DR MIKE SMITH'S
FIRST AID HANDBOOK

Dr Mike Smith is a specialist in preventative medicine and a general practitioner. He was the Chief Medical Officer of the Family Planning Association 1970–75 and their Honorary Medical Adviser 1975–90. He is an elected member of the FPA's National Executive Committee and a member of the Pet Health Council. For many years he has been a 'resident' expert guest on BBC Radio 2's *Jimmy Young Show*, LBC's *Nightline* and the medical columnist/editor for *Woman's Own*. Between 1988 and 1990 he was the expert guest on SKY TV's *Sky by Day* and continues to appear on SKY. In April 1991 he was voted the TV and Radio Doctors' 'Expert's Expert' in the *Observer* magazine's series.

He is also the author of *Birth Control*, *How to Save Your Child's Life*, *A New Dictionary of Symptoms*, *Dr Mike Smith's Handbook of Over-the-Counter Medicines*, *Dr Mike Smith's Handbook of Prescription Medicines* and the highly successful POSTBAG series.

BY THE SAME AUTHOR

**Dr Mike Smith's Handbook of
Over-the-Counter Medicines**

**Dr Mike Smith's Handbook of
Prescription Medicines**

Dr Mike Smith's Postbag series of books:
Allergies
Arthritis
Back Pain
Eating Disorders
HRT
Migraine
Skin Problems
Stress

DR MIKE SMITH'S FIRST AID HANDBOOK

Dr Mike Smith

with Sharron Kerr

Illustrations by Sally Maltby

Kyle Cathie Limited

First published in Great Britain in 1994 by
Kyle Cathie Limited
7/8 Hatherley Street
London SW1P 2QT

ISBN 1 85626 133 6

Dr Mike Smith is hereby identified as the author of this work in
accordance with Section 77 of the Copyright, Designs and
Patents Act 1988.

A Cataloguing in Publication record for this title is available from
the British Library.

Designed by Tamasin Cole
Printed in Great Britain by Cox & Wyman Ltd, Reading

CONTENTS

Acknowledgements

My grateful thanks to the Accident and Emergency Department of Queen Mary's University Hospital for their help and general comments.

PART

1

INTRODUCTION

None of us know when we'll need to react quickly to an emergency situation. And we don't know how we'll react, either, or if we'll be sure of what course of action to take. That's why a basic knowledge of first aid really is vital. It could very well turn out to be a life-saver. On four occasions, while on holiday, my wife and I have been nearby when a serious emergency has occurred and we have been able to help.

Accidents can happen so easily, and when they're least expected. Did you know that in this country more than 4000 people a year die as a result of accidents in the home? According to the Department of Trade and Industry's Consumer Safety Unit, an additional three million seek medical attention as a result of home accidents. And that doesn't take into account those people who feel their injury is not serious enough to warrant a visit to their GP or hospital.

The General Household Survey points out that the average number of home accidents treated by hospitals is 2.4 million, compared to 0.6 million from road accidents. The average number for accidents at work is 1.6 million and during sports 1.3 million. Yet where do we feel safest? At home of course!

Children are particularly vulnerable, for obvious reasons – around one child in every six visits a hospital Accident and Emergency department at some time.

From these figures you can see the need for a knowledge of first aid. Even when dealing with a minor emergency – a child burning a finger on birthday cake candles, for instance – there's

---

Accidents and over-exertion
It may seem obvious, but you are more prone to accidents if you have over-exerted yourself or are exhausted. So if at these times you can avoid driving a car, operating dangerous machinery or working at heights you should do so. It is not wimpish, just common sense!

a wrong and a right way to go about it. And if you are faced with a major emergency, knowing the right course of action to take while waiting for an ambulance can only help save lives.

The good news is that there have been successful initiatives by the Consumer Safety Unit and other bodies which have helped to reduce the number of fatalities from nearly 6000 a year in 1976 – when the Home Accident Surveillance System was introduced – to the 4000 level in 1990.

HOW YOU SHOULD REACT

If you do face a first aid crisis, remember that speed and communication are essential. Not only speed of treatment – you must also assess the situation very quickly in order to work out your list of priorities. In most instances you'll just need to use common sense.

* The first thing you should do is **keep calm** – easier said than done, I know.
* There are times when your first action must be to **dial 999** and get an ambulance to the scene as quickly as possible. These days paramedics are high-powered, highly trained professionals, able to cope with every known emergency.
* Make sure that both you and the casualty are in NO **danger**. I read recently that a man was run over twice on the motorway: once as he walked to get help and secondly when he was receiving first aid on the hard shoulder.
* You need to **judge any situation quickly.** If there is more than one casualty assess which is the most urgent. When there is more than one problem or injury, you must deal with the one that is the most serious first. As a rule of thumb it is usually more important to treat someone who is unconscious first. In times of disaster or war, professionals operate a system called 'triage'. The staff assess the situation quickly and spend time trying to save those victims that can be saved rather than letting a life slip away because they were treating a casualty who had no chance of surviving.

* **act systematically.** When faced with a casualty follow this checklist:

1 Assess the situation.
2 Ensure the safety of the casualty and all others at the scene of the accident.
3 Dial 999 to inform emergency services.
4 Deal with the most serious casualty first.
5 Check breathing and start resuscitation.
6 Stop severe bleeding.
7 Place in recovery position.
8 Give first aid to burns.
9 Check for shock, keep the casualty warm and reassure them.
10 Remember – do not move a casualty if spinal injury is suspected.

✳ Should I drive them to hospital?

I'm often asked about when you should take someone to hospital yourself rather than waiting for an ambulance to arrive. The decision really does depend on the condition of the injured person, and normally only a doctor or a qualified first-aider would be able to decide whether there is an injury to the spine which could make moving the casualty dangerous.

As a rough guide, if someone seems to be severely injured and in terrible pain (obviously suggesting broken bones), then it's best to wait for an ambulance. In the meantime, make sure the person is lying flat and is covered with a coat or anything to hand to keep them warm. When the ambulance crew arrive they will splint any broken bones, so preventing further tissue damage or shock. If there is heavy bleeding, press the area with a clean cloth, if possible, to quench the flow until help arrives.

If the pain and bleeding are not severe, and you've been warned that there may be a delay in the arrival of the ambulance, it may well be best to drive the casualty to hospital, keeping them as comfortable and as flat as possible. But an ambulance should always be called when you suspect there is spinal injury because movement could cause further damage, and the casualty may also need assistance from paramedics on the way to hospital.

WARNING

On no account move a person if a spinal injury is possible. Moving them could damage the central nervous system even further, possibly leading to paralysis. Just make sure they are safe and protected from any danger.

✽ How do you recognise life-threatening conditions?

If you look out for these three emergency situations you will be taking the first step towards saving a life:

* lack of breathing or heartbeat
* severe bleeding (when blood is pulsing out, for example)
* unconsciousness

These can occur singly or all three together. They are life-threatening because without a heartbeat the body's vital blood supply cannot be circulated and without breathing the blood won't be oxygenated so the tissues and organs will be starved of the oxygen they need in order to work. When the bleeding is severe, the body automatically shuts down all its inessential parts so that the internal organs vital for life – the brain and kidneys, for example – remain supplied. However it can't do that for long, and if bleeding continues the internal organs will stop functioning.

If someone is unconscious their head may be angled so that they don't have a clear airway. Their reflexes may also be diminished so that if they vomit their cough reflex does not work, possibly causing suffocation. Unconsciousness may also signify that the casualty is in shock and that the blood supply to the brain is starting to fail. Without urgent help it may be too late.

There's another straightforward rule you should try to remember and this is one advised by the St John Ambulance organisation. It's called the 'ABC rule' to help first-aiders remember the action they should take:

A – an open **A**irway
B – adequate **B**reathing
C – sufficient **C**irculation

Also I've found that it does help if you explain to the casualty simply and clearly what you are going to do. A child, in particular, will feel more reassured if he or she understands what is going on.

This guide is not intended to train anyone in the skills of first aid. This will only be achieved by attending a first aid course. What I do hope to do by writing this book is help you cope with any medical emergency at home, at work or at play, until professional medical help arrives or is reached. So I have included typical categories which I feel you may come across in your day-to-day life. It would be impossible in a book of this nature and size to cover every aspect of first aid, but what I have covered should help you cope in an emergency.

Hopefully, this book will also help you not to panic in a crisis and reduce the fear and anxiety surrounding illness, ill-health and accidents. I hope, too, that it answers many of the questions you might have thought of in the past and many of the questions I am regularly asked in my role as a medical broadcaster and journalist.

And, finally, I hope that this book will *discourage* people from thinking, 'It'll never happen to me,' and *encourage* them to sign up for a first aid course, because then, if it does happen to them, they'll know exactly what to do or how to help. And that can't be bad!

THE FIRST AID KIT

The aim of this book is not to get everybody worrying about the kind of accidents we could all face in our day-to-day lives. It's about being prepared and able to cope with all sorts of situations.

The first step towards coping is having a first aid kit. I believe it's essential for any home to have a well-stocked medical box. It's also useful to keep one in your car as well, and to take some form of kit on holiday with you.

Kits can be bought ready-made or you can make up your own. Make sure you keep the kit in a dry and sealable container and it must also be child-proof. If it isn't, keep it well out of a child's reach.

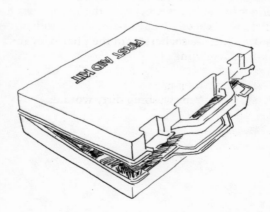

Here's a list of what I suggest you include:

* Your doctor's phone number as well as that of your nearest casualty department
* Plasters in assorted sizes
* Surgical tape
* Thermometer
* Cotton wool
* Sterile gauze dressings
* A crepe bandage
* Safety pins
* Small blunt-ended scissors
* Antiseptic solution or wipes
* Aspirin and paracetamol (paracetamol for children, too, if you have a family)
* A triangular bandage for making a sling
* An eye bath
* Calamine lotion
* Indigestion remedies
* Mineral and glucose sachets from the pharmacy for diarrhoea and vomiting
* Tweezers
* Magnesium sulphate paste
* A small bar of soap for washing dirty wounds

FIRST AID TECHNIQUES

Here are some of the important procedures you should know.

ALIVE OR DEAD?

How can you tell whether a person is dead or alive?

Your first guide will be to feel the person's pulse. This will signify if the heart is still beating. You'll also need to check for breathing which is the other sign of life. If further confirmation is needed, a doctor will look into the eye, which is a window to the blood vessels. If the blood in the retinal vessels has coagulated this is a definite indication that death has occurred.

✻ Finding the pulse

One of the most useful places to find the pulse is by pressing with two fingers on one side of the neck just below the angle of the jaw. This is called the carotid pulse. You can easily check that you have found the correct position by finding your own pulse in this area. You can also try to find the femoral pulse in the groin. These are the two best places to try in an emergency. (See also Taking a Pulse on page 21.)

✻ Check for breathing

Look for any movements in the chest or abdomen. Put an ear near the casualty's mouth or nose to try to hear any breaths. You can also hold your hand below the casualty's nostrils – you may be able to feel breath.

➕ First Aid

If there is no breath but you can still feel a pulse you'll need to give mouth-to-mouth resuscitation (see page 16). When there's no breathing as well as no pulse, you'll need mouth-to-mouth resuscitation and external heart massage (see page 13).

10

BANDAGING

Bandaging provides both a cover for a wound and a measure of support for an injured part of the body.

If you have a fully stocked first aid kit at your disposal, select the width of bandage you require. For example, you'll need a narrow bandage for a finger and a wider one, say, for an injury to a calf, and a wider one still for an abdominal problem.

It makes things easier if the casualty sits or lies down. Then you will need to support the limb on a chair, table or other hard surface if the casualty is unable to support the limb himself. This way you will have both hands free. Even the best of us can get in a tangle sometimes! When bandaging you do need to keep your hands steady – if only so as not to cause the casualty further discomfort from fumbling fingers.

A useful tip is to begin the action of bandaging below the injured area, not above. This way you can work upwards in a spiralling action. Bandages are usually sold in the form of a roll to allow easy winding movements. The free end is called the tail and the fat part of rolled bandage the head.

Get knotted

The reef knot is the best knot to use when it comes to first aid techniques. All you do is this.

1 Pass the left end over the right end and under.

2 Pass what has become the right end over what has become the left end and under.

3 Pull the two ends tight, but not too tight, because you'll want to be able to undo it again at some point.

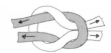

1 Hold the tail against the limb with one hand while you make the first layer of the spiral.

2 With each spiral overlap the bandage by about two-thirds. Make sure that you are not winding the bandage too tightly. If you are bandaging a finger or a toe, for example, you'll be able to tell how tight the bandage is by a darker or blueish change in colour to the skin above or below the bandage. The whole point is to protect a wound or a sprain not add to the damage by restricting blood supply!

3 Finally secure with a safety pin or tie with a reef knot (though not over a wound), by cutting the bandage down the middle, dividing it into two pieces long enough to go around the finger, wrist or leg, for instance.

✳ For an ankle

Although a bandage gives only minimal physical support to an injured ankle, it can be comforting.

1 The bandage should be anchored by holding its tail underneath the foot, and the bandage should be wrapped around the instep once.

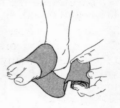

2 Then take it from the top of the instep around the back of the ankle in a figure-of-eight pattern back down and then underneath the instep again.

3 Continue in this way two or three times more, then finish by spiralling the bandage a couple of times above the ankle, and secure.

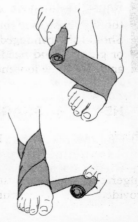

✳ For a hand

You may need to do this, for example, if you have cut your hand while preparing food.

1 Start off wrapping the bandage around the wrist, which helps keep it in place.
2 Bring the bandage across diagonally over the back of the hand, then underneath the fingers and across the palm between the finger and thumb diagonally again to the wrist.
3 Repeat this several times and secure.

✳ Bandage tubes

The art of bandaging has certainly been made much easier by the introduction of bandage tubes. These are stretched over an appropriately sized applicator which is a cylindrical-shaped 'cage'. The finger, for example, is placed into the applicator which has the bandage stretched over it. One end of the bandage is threaded on to the finger and the 'cage' is given a twist to anchor the bandage in place. The cage is then removed leaving the bandage now covering the full length of the finger. After another twist to round off at the end, the whole process is repeated to provide as many layers of tube bandage as required.

BE CAREFUL!

Whichever method you use, remember not to bandage too tightly so that you don't constrict the blood supply. Should the bandaged part later become cold or painful or get pins and needles, the bandage may be too tight and should be loosened.

HEART MASSAGE

This is required when a person's heart has stopped beating. It must be done within four minutes at the very latest, but the sooner the better really, because the brain cannot survive for longer than this without the oxygen and nutrients normally provided by the blood pumped there by the heart.

✳ For an adult

1 Put the casualty flat on his or her back. The point you need to find is where the lower ribs meet at the breast-bone.

2 Put one hand on top of your other one with arms kept straight.

3 Push down with a firm movement so that the heart is squeezed between your hands and the backbone. Because it contains many one-way valves, the heart becomes a one-way pump when squeezed, just as it does when it's beating healthily.

4 Repeat this action fifteen times quickly. The pushes should be faster than one every second – ideally 80 per minute for an adult, 100 for a child and 120 for a baby.

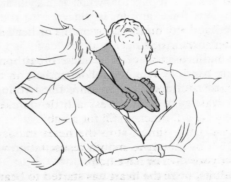

It's important to realise that the casualty won't start breathing again until the heart has started to beat. So:

5 If there are two of you, give two mouth-to-mouth breaths for every fifteen pushes to massage the heart. If you are on your own, 5 pushes to one breath (see page 16).

6 Once you feel the heart beating again check for a pulse just below the angle of the jaw on one side. Keep doing the lung inflation until you can tell the casualty is breathing again. Then roll them over on to their side in the recovery position (see page 18).

✻ For a child

Children and babies may need such resuscitation procedures if their heart stops as a result of drowning, for example,
or if they suffer a large electric shock.

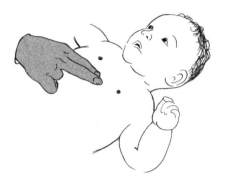

1 Lay the child gently on the floor on his or her back and
kneel down at their side.
2 Press on the lower half of the child's breastbone. Use
your whole hand, or two fingers depending on the size
of the child. Use moderate pressure for a young child
and even less for a baby. Press a little quicker than
once every second, quicker still for a baby.
3 After pressing five times, stop the heart massage and
give a breath by mouth-to-mouth resuscitation whether
you are on your own or have help.
4 As with adults, once the heart has started to beat again,
roll them into the recovery position.

A useful tip
When there's more than one of you, it can help if one person deals with the mouth-to-mouth resuscitation while
the other deals with heart massage. Keep doing this cycle
of heart massage and lung inflation until help arrives.

MOUTH-TO-MOUTH RESUSCITATION

The aim of this life-saving technique, also known as the kiss of life, is to help the casualty breathe again by giving him or her regular and persistent breaths of air from your lungs.

This technique is one of the basic and most important you can learn. It's usually used to revive someone who has stopped breathing after an accident like drowning or an electric shock. These types of accident may have only hampered the brain's ability to provoke the breathing process. If mouth-to-mouth is successful, and provided not too much time has passed since the natural breathing stopped, then the normal process should soon take over.

If the casualty is still unconscious and doesn't appear to be breathing, the heart might have stopped. Check by feeling for a pulse and if it has stopped give heart massage (see page 13) as well as mouth-to-mouth.

There really is no better way of learning this type of technique than on a first aid course. Nothing gets the message across like practising on a life-like model.

✳ Older children and adults

When a person is unconscious and seems not to be breathing, immediately begin the following procedure while someone else rings for an ambulance. (If you are on your own, shout for help.) There is no time to waste. After an accident, the airway can easily become closed, particularly when a casualty is unconscious and his or her head has rolled forward or the tongue has dropped back. Either of these factors can narrow or block the airway. The same effects can be caused by saliva or vomit in the back of the throat. So make the airway as accessible as possible.

1 Try to get the casualty flat on his or her back. Clear anything visible from the mouth using your first two fingers.
2 Bend the head back with one hand and push the jaw upwards with the other hand so that the head is tilted backwards. This lifts the tongue off the back of the throat and opens the airway.

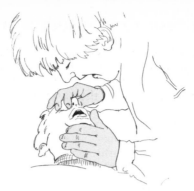

Sometimes simply opening the airway like this may help the casualty to start breathing normally again. But if not, start mouth-to-mouth resuscitation immediately:

3 Close the nostrils by pinching with your fingers.

4 Open your mouth and place it around the casualty's open mouth. It's important that your lips seal the casualty's mouth to prevent any air escaping.

5 Inhale deeply through your nose and blow vigorously into the casualty's mouth. See that the chest rises as you blow in. Then take your mouth away and let the air come out of the casualty's chest.

6 Repeat this about fifteen times a minute. Keep going until the casualty starts to breathe again. Then put them in the recovery position by turning them on to their side (see page 18).

✻ Babies

1 Place the baby on his or her back. Clear anything from the mouth and the head again needs to be tilted back very slightly (avoid tilting it too much or you may actually 'kink' the airway).

2 Place your open mouth over the baby's open mouth and nose. They are small enough for you to be able to do this and having both of the baby's airways available means that the small size of each is no handicap to the procedure.

3 Be gentle with the breath but watch to see that the chest expands as you blow into the lungs.

4 While the heart is beating and until help arrives you should carry on this artificial respiration. The very fact that the heart continues to beat after several minutes of this most likely means that you are being successful.

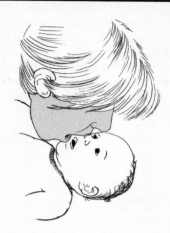

RECOVERY POSITION

If a person is unconscious and you are sure that he or she is breathing, put them on their side in the recovery position. It can be dangerous for any unconscious casualty to remain on his or her back, as the throat can be blocked by the tongue or by vomit, inhibiting breathing. The recovery position is essential because it places the head slightly lower than the rest of the body to help prevent inhalation of vomit.

The recovery position is used time and again in first aid procedures so you really should try to learn it.

WARNING

The recovery position should not be used if you suspect a spinal injury is involved.

To carry out this life-saving procedure:

1 Kneel down next to the casualty.
2 Tilt the head back and lift up the chin – this will open the airway.
3 Straighten the legs.
4 Put the arm nearest you parallel to the body with the

elbow bent, so it forms two sides of a square, and the lower arm lies across the trunk.

5 Next, bring the other arm across the chest so that the back of the hand rests against the casualty's cheek.

6 Pull the casualty towards you by gripping the thigh. The aim of this procedure is to keep the head, neck and back in a line, while the uppermost leg should be bent to stop the casualty rolling back over.

7 Now take the arm that is under the casualty and pull it out so that it's reasonably straight and parallel to the body with the palm facing upwards.

8 Then put the other arm at a right angle to the body, as shown in the diagram.

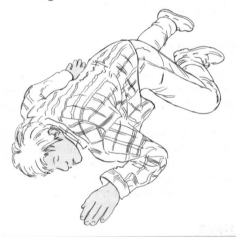

SLINGS

Slings can be used for resting injured arms or wrists, or for easing the pain of a dislocated shoulder by reducing the weight it bears.

If the hand has been injured and is painful, nature sees to it that we keep it still – or else it hurts. When our hands are held still and hanging down – by the sides of our waist, for example – they will swell. So, with an injured hand, it's important to tie the sling so that the hand is held comfortably at a higher level than the elbow. This allows gravity to keep the blood flowing freely from the hand, preventing swelling.

Slings are actually very simple to tie – but many people get themselves tangled in knots when they try to make one.

1 First get a triangular bandage. You'll need to use it with the widest angle pointing towards the elbow of the injured arm. The two narrower angles of the triangle will be used to tie a reef knot at the back of the neck.
2 Put the hand of the injured arm flat against the chest with the hand slightly raised above elbow level.
3 Place one half of the triangular bandage underneath the injured arm, putting the narrow part round the back of the neck. Then pull up the other half of the triangle to meet the bandage at the back of the neck. Tie with a reef knot (see page 11).
4 Tuck any loose edges around the elbow and secure with a safety pin.

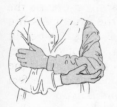
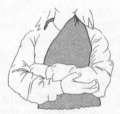
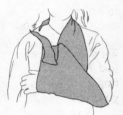

SPLINTS

If you are not fully trained in first aid you should not try to splint a broken limb. A splint is only used if the casualty has to endure a tricky journey before getting proper medical treatment, in the case of a mountain rescue perhaps. Nowadays, even if specialist help cannot reach the casualty, communications can be established and detailed instructions given.

In the absence of such help, and if a casualty has to be moved out of danger with a badly broken arm, for example, it may be best to steady the arm by bandaging it to the body to keep it immobilised and pain to a minimum. If a leg is broken, bandage it to the good leg.

STICKING PLASTERS

Can plasters slow healing? Is it better to leave a wound uncovered in order to let it 'breathe'? The purpose of applying a plaster is to keep dirt, and therefore germs, out of the wound. However, once a scab forms over an injury and it becomes dry, the body's healing process starts to lay a permanent seal just below the scab. If it then becomes soggy, germs can get a foothold.

Modern plasters are waterproof on the outside, but allow the natural moisture underneath to escape. So leaving a cut to 'breathe' was probably better advice in the past when plasters were both waterproof and airproof.

TAKING A PULSE

As I've explained under the section Alive or Dead? on page 10, in an emergency the two best places to feel for the pulse are the carotid pulse and the femoral pulse. When the urgency is not quite so great, you may prefer to try the wrist. This can be felt with the forefinger on the bone on the palm side of the wrist, just higher than the base of the thumb. It is best felt with the finger rather than the thumb because occasionally you can feel your own pulse in your thumb which could confuse you.

A regular pulse is a good indication that the heart is beating normally. No pulse signifies that the heart has stopped, and a weak or irregular pulse that it is beating inefficiently.

TEA

People who have had a fright or an emotional shock will often be offered a sweet cup of tea. This is probably because the sugar gives a burst of energy and a sense of well being, while the caffeine in the tea gives a mild 'lift' to the spirits. Sounds good to me.

The only time when it is definitely inadvisable to offer tea is if an emergency operation may be necessary. Then, nothing should be given by mouth since this could make a general anaesthetic hazardous.

TETANUS JABS

Tetanus is a serious and potentially life-threatening infectious disease which attacks the nervous system and results in acute muscle contractions particularly in the jaw and neck. The muscle spasms can get out of control, which in turn can stop breathing. Pneumonia and heart problems can also arise.

Tetanus is caused by the poison released by bacteria entering a dirty wound, particularly a deep puncture. The germs can come from soil, dirt or dust. You'd be wrong to think that tetanus is only a risk after a dog bite or severe injury. It can be caused by a small wound: for example, one suffered while gardening.

Anti-tetanus jabs are necessary because tetanus at its worst can be fatal. Even mild cases may call for five weeks' hospital treatment in an intensive care ward.

How often do we need tetanus immunisations? The threat of tetanus will always be with us. You can ask your GP or practice nurse to check when you last had a jab and whether you need a booster. Generally the tetanus vaccination should be topped up every ten years or so. So, while tetanus is serious it is comparatively rare these days – a major factor for its rarity being universal vaccination during childhood.

However, if someone cuts themselves, it's always wise to double-check with the doctor in case a further injection is necessary.

I once received a letter from a worried reader who had recently been given a booster tetanus injection. She discovered shortly afterwards that she was pregnant and was concerned that it might have harmed her baby. The tetanus injection is actually safe during pregnancy. Contrary to what many people think, a tetanus injection doesn't administer a germ – it's a toxoid. This is a substance the body's defences 'recognise' as a harmful poison – although it is in fact a false toxin. The body then makes specific antibodies against the toxoid which will be activated if you're ever infected with the real tetanus toxin.

However, as with any medicine or procedure that is undertaken just before or during early pregnancy, the important thing is that, as a mother-to-be, you feel safe. So in situations like these I would suggest talking to your GP, if only for peace of mind.

TAKING TEMPERATURES

The temperature of a patient should be taken with a clinical thermometer placed under the tongue, unless otherwise instructed. The thermometer should be shaken down to below 35°C/95°F and left under the tongue for one minute. The tongue should remain still for this time. No drinks should be given for five minutes beforehand.

Normal body temperature can range from 36–37°C/97–98.5°F, and small variations are no cause for concern. When you are taking a temperature look out for a reading of 38°C/100.4°F or over. A high temperature is usually a sign that the body is fighting infection. Coughs, colds and other infections are often accompanied by aches, pains and feverishness. Start to worry when a temperature reading is as high as 40°C/104°F – phone your doctor for advice because above this level the body's own temperature control mechanism may not be able to work effectively. You also need to consult your doctor if you have a high temperature for more than forty-eight hours, even though you have tried to lower it by self-help measures such as taking paracetamol, tepid sponging and drinking plenty of clear non-alcoholic fluids.

TOURNIQUETS

Don't use them. If an injury is spurting blood, press upon it with a clean cloth and keep pressing. As soon as possible send for someone who is fully trained and who understands the advantages and dangers of pressure points or applying tourniquets (see also page 46).

PART

2

THE A–Z OF FIRST AID

ABRASIONS AND GRAZES

An abrasion or graze differs from the term 'cut' because it involves a wound where the top layers of skin have been scraped off or rubbed away. A typical graze occurs when a child falls on the pavement or other rough surface and the skin covering the knee cap is damaged. Grazes aren't particularly serious wounds, although they can be quite painful, but they do often have small pieces of dirt or grit in them and so need careful cleansing.

✚ First Aid

One of the most germ-free items in the house is the cold water that comes from the mains tap in the kitchen – so run the wound under that when possible or, if you don't have a running mains tap, boil some water, allow it to cool to a pleasant temperature and then bathe the graze with a clean cloth.

It's important to let the air get to the wound to allow it to dry, but cover it in a way that will keep out water or dirt – and so germs – until a dry scab has formed. Depending on the part of the body affected, this is best achieved by covering with a sterile dressing or plaster bought at the local pharmacy.

Disinfectant lotions or creams can rarely improve upon the body's own antibodies and other defences, unless clean water for washing isn't available. However they do provide a hospital smell which will make you feel that the best is being done for you!

ALLERGIC REACTIONS

An allergy is the result of the body's defence mechanism going mildly haywire – reacting against substances as though they were germs. The body can also over-react when harmless substances, such as pollen in the air or pet hairs, are 'viewed' by the body's defence system (antibodies) as foreign. The antibodies in the sufferer's blood – produced to protect against germs – may then over-react to the allergen, releasing powerful chemicals which cause the symptoms of the allergy, for example a skin rash, excessive secretions in the nose or eyes, or spasm of the bronchial muscles (asthma). (Tests show that those prone to an allergy tend to have a much higher concentration of one particular type of antibody in their blood, known as immunoglobulin E – IgE for short.)

The antibodies attack our mast cells (large cells found in the skin, nose, lungs and intestines), releasing the chemical histamine and at least seven other substances which cause the tiny blood vessels (capillaries) to dilate and their walls to leak. Of course, when an infection is the cause this is good for the body as the dilated blood vessels bring in more blood cells to deal with the invaders and the secretion dilutes the infectious agent and helps to wash it out of the nose.

❶ Signs and Symptoms

An allergic reaction can take many guises. Sufferers can experience:

* difficulties in breathing
* bouts of constant sneezing
* a runny nose
* itchy eyes

Urticaria

Urticaria is a common skin problem that shows an allergic reaction has taken place. It's more often known as hives or nettle rash and it affects one in five people at some time in their lives.

Women are particularly prone, perhaps because of hormonal influences. With 'ordinary' urticaria, weals – intensely itchy raised marks on the surface of the skin – suddenly develop. They are usually short-lived, lasting for a few hours or days, but may stay longer. The weals can be any size, appear anywhere on the sufferer's body and may be numerous. They are usually pale in the middle and red around the edges and are due to dilation of the capillaries – small blood vessels under the skin – which makes their walls more permeable and enables clear fluid, called serum, to leak out. If enough serum leaks out, blisters may form.

---

* swelling of the lips, eyes or other parts of the body
* dizziness
* upset stomach
* diarrhoea
* migraine
* urticaria
* difficulties with the cardio-vascular system, causing acute shock and, if it's not treated quickly enough, even a cardiac arrest (see Anaphylactic Shock, page 30).

⊕ First Aid

If you suspect someone has had an allergic reaction the usual course of treatment is the administration of antihistamine tablets, either prescribed by your doctor or recommended by your pharmacist. These help to relieve symptoms and keep the condition under control.

For mild skin rashes or irritations, say, from insect bites or stings, try 1% hydrocortisone cream which helps to calm down any swelling and itching by cooling the skin. Ice wrapped in a wet cloth and placed on the part can also bring remarkable relief. You could apply 'wet' ice directly – but only for a few moments to avoid causing an ice 'burn'.

See also Anaphylactic Shock (page 30), Asthma Attacks (page 36), Bee Stings (page 42), Jellyfish Stings (page 155), Migraine (page 161), Wasp Stings (page 212) and Holiday First Aid (page 219).

AMPUTATIONS

Amputations can also be referred to as 'avulsion' – where limbs have been accidentally ripped off. Amputations may not necessarily involve arms or legs: accidents frequently result in a finger or toe being severed.

⊕ First Aid

When a limb, finger or toe is damaged to such an extent you will need to get emergency medical help.

Don't panic, but do shout for assistance while you get on with the first aid. It is very important to make sure that specialist help has been sent for since even the best first aider, on his own, won't have with him the intravenous fluids, the blood and the longer term life-support requirements that will be necessary!

In the meantime try to stem the flow of blood. Pressure at the site of the bleeding will stop any flow in time. The casualty will be in a great deal of pain. If shock is evident, as it almost certainly will be if the severed part is a large one, then this must be dealt with, since shock can be a killer (see page 180). It would be a tragic, wasted effort if the flow was efficiently stopped but the casualty died from shock.

Wrap any severed part in a clean cloth, if that is all there is to hand. Alternatively, in an ideal world, wrap the severed part in cling film or a clean polythene bag. If you do have ice available, crush the cubes and put them in another plastic bag or container. Then wrap the severed part in a clean cloth both to cushion it and so that the coldness of the ice doesn't damage it further. Then place it in the ice and take it to the hospital with the patient. Nowadays, it is often possible to sew it back on again.

Getting the casualty to hospital as quickly as possible is vital.

ANAPHYLACTIC SHOCK

A few people can develop an allergy to wasp or bee stings which leads to extreme, even life-threatening reactions coming on only seconds after the sting. Other people can suffer the same reaction after eating nuts, particularly peanuts.

❗ Signs and Symptoms

A sufferer may experience many, if not all, of the following:

* nausea and dizziness
* a runny, itchy nose
* watering eyes
* a sudden rash
* swelling of limbs or lips
* difficulty breathing
* they may even lose consciousness

✚ First Aid

If any of these symptoms occur after a person has been stung or unknowingly eaten a food to which they are particularly sensitive, it is essential to get them to a doctor or hospital with an Accident and Emergency unit immediately. In the meantime keep them as calm as possible, best done by retaining your composure (whatever's going on inside you!).

If someone has already had a severe allergic reaction they will probably have been prescribed an appropriate injection of adrenaline and perhaps antihistamines to carry around with them, just in case. If the reaction is particularly severe, and a doctor is available, an intravenous injection of hydrocortisone may also need to be administered.

ANGINA ATTACKS

Angina (angina pectoris) is a chest pain due to the reduction of blood flow through the coronary arteries supplying the heart muscle. Pain can also be experienced in the arm or neck, particularly on the left. It is often confused with a heart attack, but it is usually caused by a slow narrowing of the arteries: the narrower the arteries, the worse the pain. It can increase the likelihood of a heart attack, however (see page 135).

Every year some 320,000 people consult their doctor about angina. It tends to run in families and is twice as common in men. As I said, for most people the main cause of the condition is the narrowing of the coronary arteries, due to a fatty substance called atheroma laid down just below the inner lining of the coronary blood vessels. As a result, less blood is able to get to the heart muscle, and less quickly than usual too, because of the 'pinched' flow. So enough blood may still get through to

You may be interested to know that the so-called 'burn' often felt in the leg muscles during aerobic exercise is a similar reaction to that of angina and also occurs because the muscles are temporarily short of oxygen, even though the blood vessels themselves are healthy.

feed the heart during normal activity but if extra effort is asked of it – when climbing stairs, walking uphill or running for a bus, for instance – the typical gripping pain is its cry for help.

Attacks are more common in cold, windy weather and after meals. They can sometimes occur when lying flat or can even be triggered by a frightening or 'energetic' dream. Anything that increases the heart rate – such as anxiety, excitement or an over-active thyroid gland – can result in an attack. People with diabetes, high blood pressure or anaemia are also more prone to the condition. If the sufferer rests calmly, the pain usually passes after a few minutes.

❗ Signs and Symptoms

This pain is usually described as a gripping, crushing type of pain felt just behind the breastbone (and sometimes in the throat and jaw and down the arm and neck, particularly on the left), or as a tight band around the chest.

➕ First Aid

Angina symptoms can be relieved with drugs. If you suspect a person is having an attack, sit them down in their most comfortable position and make sure they take their prescribed medicine as quickly as possible. Then reassure them – sometimes holding their hand is all they'll need. Usually their stand-by medication takes effect pretty quickly. There are also

---

Angioplasty and heart bypass operations
If one of the three main coronary arteries is pinched, then angioplasty can bring remarkable relief. This technique is the blowing up of a 'balloon' in the coronary artery, which opens up the restriction so the blood can flow normally again. People can often be back at work two or three days after the operation! A heart bypass (where a blood vessel from another part of the body bypasses the artery) is an alternative surgical technique – the method chosen will depend on individual circumstances.

---

medicines available that are effective at preventing angina if taken just before any activity which might bring on an attack, such as doing the shopping or some form of exercise.

Prevention

Is an angina attack a warning to take things easy? Angina is certainly telling you that you need to change your lifestyle. There is much you can do to help yourself, which will also reduce the risk of a further heart attack. Ask your doctor for advice. Top of the list will be:

* stopping smoking (as this constricts the blood vessels)
* stopping any heavy drinking
* taking more comfortable exercise such as walking, swimming or cycling, within your tolerance level and only with medical advice
* slimming down to your ideal weight, as excess weight puts an extra strain on the heart
* resting for a while after meals
* keeping warm in winter
* not getting too worked up about things

APPENDICITIS

Appendicitis means inflammation of the vermiform (worm-like) appendix. But why do we need the appendix in the first place? It seems to have little purpose for our modern eating habits, though it does appear that certain herbivore animals, such as rabbits, find it useful.

The appendix is in fact a blind-ended tube, about the size of a little finger, which branches off the large bowel. In herbivores the appendix is much larger and therefore allows the bowels to carry and retain more digesting food than normal. It's rather like having a small reserve fuel tank!

The benefits are important for animals who eat a lot of raw plant matter, much of which contains an indigestible substance called cellulose. Because this substance can be held for a long time in the animal's bowels, the bacteria present can break it down successfully so that the animal can use it as food.

In humans, cellulose is equally indigestible and we tend to refer to it as roughage. It has the benefit of aiding the absorption of other foods and easing the work of the bowel's muscles.

The cause of appendicitis is not known. When surgeons remove an inflamed appendix, it will frequently contain remnants of food particles which are less absorbable and more inclined to pass through the bowel unchanged, like tomato pips. Consequently, it used to be suggested that these were responsible for the appendicitis. If this were true, then everyone who eats tomatoes and other seeds or nuts would get appendicitis, and, of course, they don't. Tomatoes are rich in Vitamin A and C, fibre and potassium; nuts in protein, vitamins, fibre and potassium. So I still recommend them as excellent foods.

❗ Signs and Symptoms

The main warning sign is an abdominal pain that initially waxes and wanes. It can then become intense and localised in the lower right-hand side of the abdomen. Touching or applying pressure to that area will definitely make the pain worse.

Loss of appetite, nausea and occasionally vomiting are other symptoms, as are a slightly raised temperature. There may also be diarrhoea or constipation, and the person may have bad breath and their mouth feel unpleasant.

The symptoms of an acute appendix can develop between four and forty-eight hours after the appearance of the first symptoms. The main sign is pain that occurs in waves, tending to start around the navel and moving to a point (known as

Grumbling appendix
Some older readers may have been told in the past that they had a 'grumbling appendix'. About thirty years or so ago abdominal pains of one sort or another were put down to this condition, but that's not thought to be the case any more. What used to be symptoms associated with a grumbling appendix are now thought to have been symptoms of irritable bowel syndrome. These days if an appendix is definitely thought to be inflamed it will be taken out.

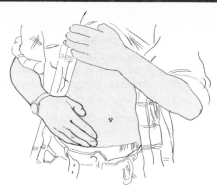

McBurney's point) below the right of the navel on a line between the pubic bone and the bony prominence on the top part of the pelvic girdle. McBurney's point is tender when pressed and also usually when the pressure is released. Doctors call the latter 'rebound tenderness' and it is due to the infected appendix inflaming the lining membrane of the abdomen (the peritoneum).

Should the appendix burst, the infected matter will inflame a wide area of the peritoneum, causing peritonitis. If this happens, there will be a stiffening in the patient's abdominal muscles and they will also probably have a rapid pulse, shallow breathing and clammy skin.

✚ First Aid

If someone is suffering from these symptoms seek medical help as soon as possible. As a safeguard you shouldn't give them anything to eat or drink, just in case they will need emergency surgery and therefore a general anaesthetic. If the patient is very thirsty he or she can take small amounts of water to rinse the mouth and make it feel less dry. Don't give any painkillers or other medication.

There's not much you can do once an inflamed appendix is diagnosed, except give the sufferer tender loving care and talk quietly and comfortingly to them until they are taken to the operating theatre.

Our bodies do not seem to miss the appendix once it has been removed and the site has been cleaned up nicely by the surgeon. Uncommonly, when the area has been particularly inflamed, debris left by the oozing of the appendix may cause pieces of bowel or other tissue to stick together. These adhesions can interrupt the free movement of the bowel and, where there is severe pain and other abdominal symptoms, a surgeon may have to perform a 'freeing' operation later on.

ASTHMA ATTACKS

Asthma is an inflammatory condition that causes a swelling of the lining membrane of the breathing tubes, thus constricting them. At the same time, the very small muscles in these tubes contract, narrowing them even further.

In Britain, about 2000 people a year die, and some end up brain-damaged, as a result of a serious asthma attack. More than one in ten of us suffer from some kind of asthma – and it does seem to be on the increase. No one really knows why, though some argue that specialists are simply spotting it more often. Other experts believe that the increase in air pollution – mainly from cars – could be a cause.

The most common cause of asthma attacks is an allergy, usually to house-dust mites, pollen or animals. Chest infections can also trigger asthma. In adults, attacks are not necessarily caused by an allergy, but by one of many other triggers such as an over-reaction of the lung-lining tissues to cold temperatures, for example, or to exercise. In someone who suffers from asthma, worry and anxiety, perhaps caused by pressure at work or at home, can make the condition worse.

A friend of mine who has a son with severe asthma always told him to retain two small coins in one particular pocket so that he could phone her from wherever he was when he knew a bad attack was coming on and she would collect him. It's as well she suggested two coins. When he first felt the need to phone, all his mother heard were very deep breaths – the poor little chap couldn't even get a word out. She thought he was a heavy breather and put the phone down on him, only realising as she did so who it was. Thankfully he managed to get the next coin in and she went to his aid!

Asthma is surprisingly common and can be treated readily and effectively. If diagnosed, your doctor will probably prescribe an inhaler. Medicines are given to help prevent the symptoms occurring or to give relief – or both. The medicines used to treat asthma include bronchodilators (airway openers) and inhaled steroids to help dampen down the inflammation and irritability of the airways.

⏸ Signs and Symptoms

Symptoms may be one or any of the following:

* chest 'tightness'
* shortness of breath
* a wheeze or a cough

These are worse at some times more than others because the swelling of the lining tissues waxes and wanes throughout the day. Consequently the obstruction of airflow is variable – and it is this variation which is the main characteristic of asthma.

The symptoms of a severe attack can also include:

* a severe shortness of breath – often the patient will seem to be fighting to breathe
* paleness in the face
* an inability to speak, as well as exhaustion

⊕ First Aid

The basic aim of dealing with an asthma attack is obviously to help the sufferer breathe more easily again.

In a severe attack you'll need to seek medical assistance by calling an ambulance immediately. While you're waiting for the ambulance to arrive, try to get the sufferer to take his or her medication, which should help ease any wheezing. They'll have been told how to take it and how often. If, in their respiratory distress, they are barely able to speak – not at all uncommon in a severe attack – accept their refusal to partake in any suggestions as it may only make them more agitated if they don't have the breath to explain their reasons.

Another action you can take is to help the sufferer into a comfortable position, for example sitting up in a chair with their hands on their knees, perhaps leaning slightly forward. They will usually do this instinctively, as by so doing they are unconsciously anchoring their top ribs and so allowing the secondary muscles of respiration around the neck to be used to their best effect.

A severe asthma attack can be extremely frightening so you'll need to appear calm (even if you're frightened too) until help arrives.

When an attack isn't so serious the sufferer still needs to take his or her medicine as soon as possible. If the attack doesn't respond to the usual treatment you must seek your doctor's advice.

Prevention

People with asthma have airways which have become over-sensitive. So if you suffer from asthma and know what triggers an attack, do obviously try to avoid that trigger. Your doctor is likely to have told you to do some or all of the following:

* keep your house as free from dust as possible
* undertake moderate exercise, especially children, even though exercise can sometimes trigger an attack. Using a bronchodilator drug beforehand helps to prevent an attack. Most asthmatics find that swimming is a helpful form of exercise
* always keep your drugs close at hand
* always take your anti-inflammatory inhalations as instructed. These will usually be steroids and they are remarkably effective at preventing an attack.

If you feel your asthma is getting worryingly worse, you should follow your doctor's instructions – often now printed as treatment guidelines and given to sufferers or their carers as soon as the diagnosis has been made. But when in doubt, contact your doctor.

BACK INJURIES

Most back pains are due to strains, sprains and tears. This is because the small muscles supporting the spine work at a disadvantage. To hold us upright they have to be tense most of the time. A sudden extra twist or strain and the muscles, tendons or their bony attachments give way, causing the symptoms.

When you encounter your first attack of back pain, or if the pain is severe and you are in a great deal of discomfort which doesn't ease after a day, I would advise you to see your GP before trying any DIY treatments. He may be able to determine straightaway if you are suffering from a back problem and not a symptom of another condition such as a kidney complaint.

✚ First Aid

The treatment of back pain usually involves:

* immobilisation
* rest
* the relief of pain

* Pain relief

It is important to administer pain relief quickly to prevent further discomfort. Aspirin and other non-steroidal anti-inflammatory drugs like ibuprofen, which alleviate pain as well as reducing stiffness and inflammation, can be helpful.

Ibuprofen is a popular option when it comes to dealing with back pain. It's thought to work by blocking the enzyme needed for the production of prostaglandins, which pass on pain signals to the brain. Prostaglandins also cause swelling, which makes you feel even worse and can inhibit movement.

Ibuprofen is also available in a gel form (for example, one brand name is Ibuleve) so that you can apply it directly at the point of pain, where it is quickly absorbed into the skin. It's claimed to be particularly useful for backache, and can be applied up to three times a day. However ibuprofen isn't recommended for patients with a history of kidney problems, stomach conditions, asthma or aspirin-sensitivity, without the advice of their doctor. It also shouldn't be taken while pregnant or while breastfeeding.

Painkillers

To be most effective, over-the-counter painkillers need to be taken at regular intervals, according to the instructions on the packet. By taking these painkillers regularly a constant level of relief is maintained in the bloodstream and consequently pain is prevented from resurfacing.

But with any painkiller, don't take it for more than a few days, unless your doctor has told you otherwise. Don't think that by taking a lot of painkillers in one go they'll work better. Never exceed the stated dose – overdoses can be dangerous. And whatever you do, don't mix and match painkillers. Always consult your doctor or pharmacist before taking an over-the-counter medicine if you are already on medication or have a medical condition.

Paracetamol is an effective painkiller, too, but it won't help reduce any inflammation.

✳ Massage

If you're averse to taking tablets you'll be pleased to know that massaging the affected area of your back or painful muscle can be soothing. You don't have to use a vibrator, linament or muscle rub, although there are plenty on the market.

✳ Rest

The injured part needs a period of rest while healing gets underway, followed by a further period of gentle exercise and rehabilitation. Research has shown, however, that staying in bed for too long can make the problem worse, because the muscles of the body quickly lose their tone – immediate strength – when they remain unexercised. This process can happen within a few days, causing the sufferer to feel very weak when he or she first gets out of bed. The muscles around the vertebrae work under the greatest mechanical difficulty, so if they lose their tone, the back is further disadvantaged, over and above the condition that caused the sufferer to take to his or her bed in the first place.

Some experts believe that sufferers should get up and start

moving about as soon as the pain eases enough to be able to do so. Spending too much time in bed can also be bad for your circulation. Ideally, if you consult your GP he or she can arrange physiotherapy treatment from the very start.

So, if you have to rest in bed most therapists will advise that you move around gently and without discomfort from time to time, changing position or even just wriggling your toes; rotate your ankles in a clockwise direction then back again, and raise and lower your knees several times if you can (provided you haven't been told not to).

BED SORES

If someone who is confined to bed is so ill or paralysed that they can't turn over, they risk developing painful bed sores. The skin can crack and weep and, as a result of the continuous pressure on a certain part of the body, the tissues below the skin can become lifeless and quickly 'wear away'. These painful areas of skin are also known as pressure sores and usually appear on the buttocks, heels and elbows due to pressure and friction from the bed itself.

The problem arises because the pressure prevents an adequate amount of blood getting through to supply the tissue with oxygen and nutrients. This doesn't happen in healthy people because the normal sensations of discomfort – which at their worst become pins and needles – make us turn over or move about, even in our sleep.

Elderly people who have to stay in bed because of illness are particularly vulnerable. Often their skin is not as supple or resilient as it used to be and their ageing nerves are less sensitive to the warning signals that their skin and tissues are becoming numb.

✚ First Aid

Barrier creams, zinc and castor oil cream or petroleum jelly, used frequently and rubbed in well, can help protect the skin from irritation, as can talcum powder. It is the regular rubbing that is important. In hospital, when there is a likelihood of such sores developing, the nursing staff will treat the vulnerable areas every four to six hours, and turn the patient every two hours.

Should the skin look particularly sore or, even worse, if it starts to weep, seek help from your doctor or a registered nurse immediately. Once a bed sore has started, it will need regular nursing attention several times a day to clear it up.

🔆 Prevention

The less a patient moves around, the more likely bed sores are to develop. So, if you're looking after an elderly person who is confined to bed, make sure he or she changes position as often as possible, and help them to do so if necessary.

BEE STINGS

For most people a sting is a painful and sometimes embarrassing experience – my face once swelled up after I was stung on my top lip by a bee that was immersed in my drink.

A bee will sting only as a last resort, as it leaves its sting behind and dies soon afterwards.

✚ First Aid

Remove the sting with a fingernail by scraping it out sideways and in the direction the sting is pointing, rather than pinching and pulling it out, as this can squeeze the remaining venom into the skin. Another method is to scrape the blunt side of a knife along the skin's surface to squeeze the venom out.

In the case of a bee sting, symptoms such as pain, swelling,

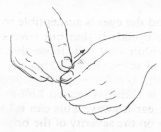

or a hot, red, swollen area of skin, are the result of the body's reaction to the poison. To counteract acid in a bee sting, apply ice-cold water containing a little bicarbonate of soda.

For stings in the mouth, multiple stings or if a child under the age of two is stung, it is best to seek medical advice without delay. Stings in the mouth can cause swelling to such a degree that it could block airways and consequently endanger life. With young children this is even more dangerous as their airways are smaller and narrower, so they are more at risk of suffocation.

If you swallow a bee there's not a lot you can do. If you have a known hyper-sensitivity then you should alert your doctor and give yourself the shot of adrenaline with which you have been provided (see Anaphylactic Shock, page 30). If you are not sensitive to bee stings then it is probably wise to notify your doctor as a safeguard.

Prevention

To avoid being stung it's useful to remember:

* not to use perfume, hair sprays or aftershave when bees or wasps are around, as they can be attracted by the scent
* to examine food and sweet drinks before putting them in your mouth and wipe food off your lips if eating out of doors
* not to panic if bees or wasps buzz around you, and don't hit out at them – just ignore them or walk away.

BLACK EYES

The delicate area around the eyes is susceptible to easy bruising because the skin of the eyelids is thin but covers several quite large veins which lie within very soft, loose tissue. This tissue will readily fill with blood at the slightest knock.

The range of colours experienced is the result of the body's cleaning process, which converts leaked blood into different chemicals in order to clear it away. This can take some two to three weeks, depending on the severity of the bruising.

WARNING

If you experience problems with your vision after a blow to the eye, consult your doctor.

⊕ First Aid

An ice pack, a cold compress or a packet of frozen peas wrapped in a clean, damp cloth should be placed over the eye area as soon as possible (applying the packet directly could damage the skin further).

What about a pound of your butcher's best steak, which seems to be everyone's first line of treatment? I think this has become a traditional remedy because it's cold, it's wet and it's malleable, moulding easily to the form and shape of that area of the body. A clean, well wrung out flannel which has been soaked in cold water will work just as well, as long as the flannel is squeezed sufficiently beforehand to prevent any water from entering the eye. It won't cost as much either and you can feel happy about using it again!

BLEEDING, INTERNAL

Internal bleeding can follow an injury or signify the presence of a medical condition. It's dangerous simply because you don't know how much bleeding is involved or when it has stopped, and the person may go into shock at any moment.

In fact, the first occurrence of any unusual blood from any orifice of the body is worth a medical consultation. You'll need to get a doctor's help to ascertain the cause and therefore minimise any damage.

⊕ Signs and Symptoms

Signs of internal bleeding include:

* blood loss from the vagina in between periods, particularly after sexual intercourse – referred to as inter-menstrual and post-coital bleeding
* passing blood with urine (see page 49)

* anal bleeding (Small spots of fresh red blood after passing a hard stool following constipation shows that you might have a tear or an abrasion of a pile. But should there be any anal bleeding when you have opened your bowels, involving a lot of red blood, or altered blood which is darker in colour (like runny black tar) and represents a bleed higher up the digestive system, there is more cause for concern.)
* coughing up blood (this will usually be bright red in colour)
* vomiting blood (If a blood vessel bursts in the lining of the stomach, for example if a peptic ulcer has caused it to erode, blood will often be vomited up. If it is due to a sudden large bleed this will usually be bright red. If it is due to a slower seepage of blood, which the digestive juices have started to break down, it will be more like small brown granules.)
* bleeding from the ear (this usually signifies that the eardrum has been perforated – unless the person has recently had a blow to the head, when it could signify a small fracture of the skull)

As well as the obvious signs of blood, look out for:

* a weakening of the casualty's pulse
* cold clammy skin
* internal pain
* the casualty may look pale and rather grey – in short, be in shock, a dangerous condition (see page 180).

✚ First Aid

When internal bleeding is likely to be present, call an ambulance.

In the meantime reassure the patient that help is on its way and ask them to lie down with their legs slightly raised and their feet supported on pillows (or anything that is handy). You need to raise the legs to prevent shock developing. If it's cold, cover the patient and if he or she becomes unconscious, put them in the recovery position (see page 18) as quickly and gently as possible.

BLEEDING FROM WOUNDS

When dealing with bleeding bear in mind that even large arteries that have been damaged will eventually cease to bleed if firm pressure is applied. So don't panic.

Also remember that when dealing with blood or body fluids care should be taken, where possible, to avoid direct contact (see pages 234–5).

✚ First Aid

For minor bleeding, press firmly on the wound using a pad of clean cloth, if there's any to hand. If not, use your fingers. Keep pressing until the bleeding stops.

Severe bleeding should be dealt with promptly but calmly. The casualty needs to be taken to the nearest hospital with an Accident and Emergency unit. Initially the procedure is the same as dealing with less severe bleeding: cover the wound with a clean (sterile, if at all possible) pad of cloth and again press down firmly to staunch the flow. You may need to ask the casualty to lie down in a position in which they feel comfortable and raise the wounded limb as high as possible. This allows the pressure of gravity to help reduce the bleeding. Support a limb with one hand and press on the wound with the other. If the pad becomes soaked in blood quickly get another, or just keep pressing anyway.

✹ Do not use a tourniquet

Use only pressure to stem the flow of blood – on no account use a tourniquet. Too often in the past these have unwittingly been tied too tightly, and the part affected has been lost because its blood supply was cut off for too long. Tourniquets cut off the total supply to a limb instead of stopping just the bleeding of the injured area. Sometimes, too, a tourniquet has been applied which, though not tight enough to stop the blood going through the artery (which is at a higher pressure), is tight enough to stop the blood in the vein (at a lower pressure) from returning – so causing an increase in bleeding. And a muscle that has been starved of blood for too long can subsequently swell within its tough fibrous and unstretchable sheath, crushing itself in the process and causing a condition known as Crush Syndrome. This in itself can be life-threatening (see page 82).

It is rarely necessary to apply pressure at the point of the main artery, where blood to a limb can be stopped completely. Known as pressure points, where such an artery runs over a bone, the blood supply can be easily 'turned off' by pressing upon them. Such 'points' are the brachial point where the pulse in the brachial artery can be felt as it passes down the inside of the upper arm, and the femoral point where the femoral artery pulse can be felt in the centre of the groin on either side. In both these places the artery runs against a bone so firm pressure can be easily applied. But it is rarely wise to do this. Pressure on these points is likely to be justified only when the whole limb has been severely injured or lacerated, or the person applying the pressure has been fully trained and is able to assess the effects against the disadvantages.

The main disadvantage is that if, incorrectly, the blood supply is cut off for too long the limb may never recover and so become gangrenous. It may then have to be surgically removed.

BLINDNESS, SUDDEN

The sudden loss of all or part of a person's sight – for example unexplained blurring of vision – should be treated as a medical emergency.

If it is unrelated to an injury it could be caused by a migraine, acute glaucoma, acute inflammation of the optic nerve or the tissues within the eye (which are known as the uveal tract), a thrombosis of, or bleeding from, an artery, or retinal detachment. (It will not usually be a symptom of a brain tumour, although this needs to be considered.) It will often be accompanied by symptoms related to the condition in general – one-sided head pain in migraine, for example – but may uncommonly occur as the main symptom.

You need to contact a doctor at once or get the patient to a hospital with an Accident and Emergency unit.

BLISTERS

A blister is a 'bubble' of fluid in the skin caused by rubbing or burning. The bubble formation is probably a defence to protect the skin beneath.

✚ First Aid

Wash the foot, cover the blister with a non-stick, light, sterile dressing at night and a plaster that is waterproof yet allows the skin to breathe during the day. If the blister starts to feel very painful and hot, and looks red and swollen, it's become infected and the patient will need to see a doctor.

You shouldn't prick blisters because you could be poking germs and a potential infection through the breach in the skin. Often blisters break of their own accord, which lets out fluid while leaving a covering over the raw area of skin. If the blister is causing so much discomfort that you feel you must prick it, wash the blister first, then use a sterile needle. But it really is best to leave it alone.

Sometimes the blister will not burst and the fluid will be absorbed back into the body while the germ-tight cover remains intact.

⊘ Prevention

Occasionally I receive a letter from someone who is about to go on a walking holiday for the first time and who would like to know how to prevent blisters! This depends on the careful buying and preparation of footwear.

Many hardened walkers have their own preferences for boots or shoes, foot care and the thickness of socks, but my advice is this – buy and get used to your footwear well before your proposed holiday in order to break in the shoes/boots. Then start walking short distances, gradually increasing the length, until you're sure any discomfort has been overcome. The top layers of the skin will naturally thicken and harden when prepared in this way.

BLOOD IN URINE

Blood in the urine should always be investigated by a doctor, because if the patient hasn't had an accident or there are no signs of obvious injury, it may imply various problems. Causes could be an infection, or a papilloma (warts) in the bladder, for example. If untreated, warts can spread or bleed heavily and are sometimes malignant, though early treatment can cure them completely.

The patient may need to be referred to a specialist, a urologist, who may advise a cystoscopy – looking at the inside of the bladder through a thin, illuminated, flexible tube passed up the urine tube – urethra – under a light anaesthetic. So, even if the patient feels well, it is essential to establish the cause of any bleeding.

BOILS, BURSTING

A boil – sometimes called a furuncle – is usually due to a bacterial infection of the skin and is extremely painful. It usually starts in and around a hair follicle where skin cells are destroyed by bacteria. Pus then develops, building up such pressure that the boil can burst, requiring treatment as below.

If boils recur, do consult a doctor. They will usually be due to no more than a particularly virulent strain that has 'settled in' and may need a prescription of antibiotics to shift it. Bacteria nest in the warm, moist areas of the body, like the cleavage between the legs, so frequent hand and bottom washing is important. These germs can be dabbed around the body by our hands without even realising it and this may be all that's required to cause an infection.

Occasionally, though, there may be an excess of sugar in the bloodstream which is causing the germs to stay with you and your doctor may decide to test for diabetes, which can be one reason for boils recurring.

➕ First Aid

If a boil does burst, just clean the area with plenty of cooled boiled water or clean mains tap water. Or, if you prefer, try an antiseptic wipe or piece of cotton wool moistened with an antiseptic solution – but do follow the instructions on the packaging. Then apply a clean, dry dressing which will need to be changed frequently. Pain can be relieved with painkillers. Ask your pharmacist for advice on a suitable product.

BREATHING DIFFICULTIES

Breathing difficulties can become life-threatening. They can range from simply noisy breathing after a cold or other chest infection, to the wheeziness of asthma (see page 36) through to choking due to an obstruction (see page 68). Severe breathing difficulties in children can be diagnosed as croup (see page 81).

Breathing problems that are accompanied by a high temperature can be dangerous, particularly for the elderly, and suggest the presence of a chest infection such as bronchitis or pneumonia. Sudden attacks of difficult breathing with the coughing up of phlegm or blood will need medical investigation.

Over-breathing can be a sign of hyperventilation due to anxiety (see page 173) and fume inhalation can also cause breathing problems (see page 123).

Painful breathing can suggest there is a problem affecting the lungs and their covering membranes – the pleura – just under the chest wall.

If the patient suffers breathing difficulties and a chest pain, there may be a problem affecting the heart. So any unusual and extreme difficulty with breathing, particularly when accompanied by a blueish tinge around the mouth, must be treated as a medical emergency requiring immediate help.

✚ First Aid

If the casualty has stopped breathing then you must start emergency resuscitation procedures at once (see Mouth-to-Mouth Resuscitation, page 16). And if anyone else is nearby, get them to call an ambulance.

BROKEN BONES

If you suspect someone has a broken bone you need to proceed with great care because you don't want to cause any extra damage. Broken bones will always need proper medical attention and usually an X-ray to determine the exact nature and extent of the fracture.

The skeleton is made up of more than 200 bones. There are twenty-nine bones in the skull, twenty-six in the foot and twenty-seven in the hand, for example. So you can see the potential for fractures is immense.

❗ Signs and Symptoms

You should consider that a bone or bones may be broken if there has been a serious accident and the casualty is unconscious, or in great pain, or unable to move a limb for themselves.

If a limb is out of the line of its usual flexing ability – a leg or arm bent sideways, for example – then of course the injury is obvious. But it's rarely that straightforward.

Severe and immediate swelling and pain in the affected part is also a very good guide. Blood coming from any orifice in the skull – mouth, nose, ears or eye sockets – suggests a skull fracture, as does fluid (from the spine) coming from the ears or nose.

You should be suspicious of broken bones after any fall suffered by an elderly person, however trivial it may seem, and by a younger person if they can't or don't want to get up due to pain, even though at first sight you consider they should be able to.

X-rays

X-rays produce images of the body's bones, organs or internal tissues through the medium of radiography. This uses carefully controlled electromagnetic radiation to get an image on a photographic plate or a fluorescent screen. Bone tissue gives the clearest X-ray picture.

X-rays are not carried out during pregnancy – especially in its early phases – to avoid radiation damage to the more susceptible cells of the growing baby.

✳ Types of Fracture

There are four main types of fracture:

* greenstick – a break that is not complete
* simple – a clean break but the skin surrounding the bone is not broken
* compound – a compound fracture involves broken bone and a rupturing of the skin nearby
* comminuted – which involves the bone being shattered into tiny fragments

✚ First Aid

Do not move any casualty with a suspected fracture unless:

* you are sure that the part affected can be immobilsed and supported so that it can't be damaged further
  OR
* the person is in a dangerous area – for example, on a motorway at night – and then only with extreme care.

Great care is especially important if you think the casualty has injured his or her spine or neck. A clumsy move under these conditions can further or permanently damage the central nervous system, rendering the casualty paralysed from that point downwards.

It's useful to keep the person still and warm, if needs be, by covering them with a blanket or coat. You really shouldn't try to deal with broken bones unless you are qualified to do so. If the casualty is in no immediate danger and is comfortable, it's far better to leave it to the trained professionals. Don't give the casualty a drink in case they need an operation.

I stress again, if you have to move the casualty for safety reasons be very gentle. With a broken leg you should secure the injured limb to the leg that's all right before moving the person. Put some form of padding between the legs and at the ankles and knees. Gentle immobilisation needs to be used for all limb fractures. With a broken arm, the arm needs to be padded against and supported by the trunk, held there by wide strips of cloth fastened as temporary bandages.

WARNING
Don't give someone with a suspected fracture anything to eat or drink. They may need corrective surgery and therefore a general anaesthetic.

Here are some typical fractures and the warning signs that might imply the area is damaged. Very often the casualty will have heard the bone 'crack'.

* Broken ankle
Look out for shock (see page 180), swelling, pain and the casualty's stated inability to move the ankle joint. Don't ask them to move it and tell them not to if you're concerned that it might be fractured.

* Broken arm
The arm may look unusual – for example, where the fore-arm should be straight, it now looks curved. It may be impossible for the casualty to hold anything in his or her hand. There will be swelling, pain and tenderness.

* Broken cheekbone
Look for swelling and blood coming from the nose and mouth. A large black eye may quickly develop. A cold, wet, clean cloth held against the eye may contain its enlargement. Occasionally, the bone may move as the person breathes in and out. Seek urgent medical attention.

* Broken collar-bone
The collar-bone (clavicle) lies between the shoulder and the top of the breastplate in the front and top of the chest.

A collar-bone can be fractured as a result of indirect force, i.e. not caused by a direct hit but by undue pressure on another part of the body. An example would be when a person slips and reaches out with their hand to break the fall – the arm may remain intact but the collar-bone could fracture.

A sling should be used to support the weight of the arm and remind the patient that he shouldn't use that arm. Under these conditions, the collar-bone will heal in six to eight weeks, but do seek professional medical help.

✻ Broken finger

A sudden flip sideways while participating in a vigorous sport may fracture a finger or pull its joint tendons out of the bone's anchor points. A common injury is the knuckle of the little finger when the fist doesn't land properly during a fall, or even a punch! Depending on the severity, most finger fractures can be immobilised by splinting them against the next finger.

✻ Broken jaw

The jaw will be very painful and difficult to move. The teeth can become misplaced as a result of a blow, or there may be a cut on the inside of your mouth together with the swelling, tenderness and bruising that accompanies most fractures.

A large bandage or scarf used as a sling under the jaw to support it and tied on the top of the head will immobilise it for transport to the Accident and Emergency department.

✻ Broken nose

When a nose has received a blow and is obviously swollen or out of alignment, medical attention is needed. While you are waiting for help, soak a clean cloth or flannel in cold water. Wring it out well and then apply to the painful area. If there's a nose bleed, you'll need to deal with that as well (see page 169). Sometimes a doctor will have to elevate the bones and cartilages to achieve a satisfactory cosmetic result.

✻ Broken leg

A fracture can make the leg look crooked or twisted and swollen. The casualty may not be able to put any weight on that limb without experiencing severe pain.

A fracture of the thigh (the femur) is very likely to cause shock, as sometimes it may leak several pints of blood into the soft tissues of the thigh before anyone realises what's happening. My advice is to regard any thigh fracture as a 'shocking' experience and treat for shock, whether it appears to be present or not (see page 180).

✻ Broken pelvis

In the elderly, a broken pelvis can be caused by simply tripping down a few stairs. Because their bones are often quite

Chipped bones
What's the difference between a chipped bone and a broken bone? Well, there's no difference. A chip means just what it says, the break involves one tiny chip and one big bit. A chip is a fracture and so more often than not is treated in the same way.

brittle such a simple fall can lead to fractures. It can also be the consequence of an awkward fall (as in skiing) or a crush injury (as in a car crash).

Signs of a broken pelvis may include severe pain when the casualty tries to walk or put weight on their legs. There can be tenderness and discomfort around the pelvic area – the lower abdomen and lower back – and shock can develop. Passing urine may be difficult, or even impossible as in some instances – when the fracture is more severe and the bones are out of alignment – other nearby organs or structures are damaged, causing as many problems as the break itself. For example, if the pelvis is broken at the front, it can tear the closely attached soft tissues, such as the bladder and its drainage tube, the urethra. Extra care and specialist attention will be needed to bring about the repair of such a vital structure.

And, similarly, should a fracture that is a break rather than just a crack become unaligned, this can affect the hip – so an orthopaedic surgeon's skills may be required to fix the pieces together so that the patient will have a mobile hip again once it's healed.

For many people, a broken pelvis (just like a crack in a bone in any other part of the body) is likely to cause a continuing dull, aching pain. It is nature's way of telling us that the part concerned requires rest so that it has a chance to heal.

An ambulance should be called as soon as possible. In the meantime, make the casualty more comfortable – advise him or her to lie on their back with their knees bent or straight – whichever is the least painful. This will usually take the strain off the pelvis. They should keep their legs still. You may be able to bandage the legs together, perhaps with a scarf tied around the ankles, but don't do this if it triggers additional pain.

Immediate immobility allows the bone to begin to knit

together – a process that is extremely fragile and susceptible to damage. Resting increases the blood supply to the injured part, thus bringing extra oxygen and nutrients to aid the activity of the repair cells which lay down fibres and cartilage, a soft fore-runner to bone. For the majority of pelvic injuries, rest, time and sometimes painkillers are all that are needed to allow the fracture to heal.

✳ Broken wrist

When someone falls they instinctively hold out their hand. This can lead to a broken wrist as it takes the full force of the fall. Commonly this results in a Colles' fracture, where the fore-arm bones are broken just above the wrist. Another break which may not be immediately apparent is a fracture of a wrist bone at the base of the thumb – the scaphoid.

With a Colles' fracture the wrist will be out of alignment, making the diagnosis straightforward, but with a scaphoid frac-ture there may be little to see. It's also sometimes difficult for a lay person to know the difference between a sprain and a frac-ture. There could be swelling, for instance, in both cases. Pain, the type of injury – that is, if the fracture is an open one with bone protruding – how the casualty fell and the presence of shock are the strongest clues. The classic Colles' fracture occurs when someone falls heavily on an outstretched palm of the hand.

If you think someone has broken their wrist, tie on a sling to support the injured arm before transfer to hospital.

Getting plastered

Don't be too surprised if a broken arm, for example, is not put in plaster. Fractures aren't always treated in this way – it depends which bone is broken and where. One of the most common bone fractures, which doesn't require more than a sling to allow healing to take place, is the fracture of a collar-bone (see page 53). Likewise, if there's a hairline fracture at the edge of another bone in the arm, but the bone isn't out of alignment and isn't interfering with a joint, the arm need only be rested in a sling.

✳ Rib fractures

Rib fractures can be the result of a car accident, a fall or a knock. They are quite different from other bone breaks. Each rib lies in its own fibrous sheath so the ribs can break while remaining 'splinted' by their own sheaths. When this happens, no treatment is necessary other than painkillers. There is likely to be pain around the chest which worsens on breathing in. There may be an open wound and there may also be signs of internal bleeding (see page 44).

With a simple rib fracture, most of the pain and unpleasant symptoms go in about a month, although some pain can still be felt for another month or two. After that, the rib is virtually as good as new.

During the days following the accident, the bone repair-cells interweave strong fibres which anchor the surfaces together and, finally, the bone-producing cells turn the whole area – called a callus – into firm bone. Throughout this time, such perfect remodelling is taking place that, particularly in a young person, an X-ray taken a year or so later may not be able to detect that a fracture ever occurred.

Unfortunately, in later life, a fracture can cause aches and pains and, in particular, arthritis when it has interfered with the workings of a joint.

BRUISES

A bruise can develop as a result of a knock, tear or even a strain, provided it's severe enough, and is caused by blood leaking from damaged blood vessels and then spreading into surrounding tissue. The leaked blood is converted into different chemicals as it is broken down by the body's clearing-away process, which explains the range of colours.

Some women find they bruise more easily, and sometimes quite severely, just before their period. As the cause of a bruise is a knock resulting in bleeding into the tissues, excessive bleeding would imply that the blood is failing to clot or that the small blood vessels around the injured area break more easily than usual.

> *Bruised bones*
> Can bones become bruised? I'm often asked. Yes, blood
> can be, and often is, lost into them at the time of an
> injury. The body's scavenging mechanism will clear it
> away eventually.

There is an old wives' tale that the blood fails to clot as
quickly as usual at period time because nature is preparing to
'thin' the blood so the menstrual flow will run more freely.
There's no medical explanation why women should bruise
more easily at this time, and I happen to believe that the old
wives were right, though there is no measurable proof.

✱ Contusions
What's the difference between a bruise and a contusion?
Not a lot. A contusion is usually so called when the swelling
hasn't been discoloured by leaking blood, suggesting that tissue
fluid is escaping instead. The treatment is the same.

✱ Haematomas
A haematoma is the name given to a leak of blood into the
tissues which occurs quickly and is then able to 'pool' – collect
in one place. It will usually have the same symptoms as a
bruise. Rarely it may need to be drained, through a syringe, by
a doctor.

➕ First Aid
Don't rub or massage the bruised area – pressure may
make things worse. Bruises are particularly painful if they lie
over a bone as here the clogged tissues are more tightly
stretched. An ice pack, in the form of a cold compress or a
packet of frozen peas wrapped in a damp towel (peas are very
useful for first aid because the packet moulds easily to the shape
of your body), applied immediately after the knock, may help to
reduce the bruising; it may also help to numb the pain afterwards.
If a leg is bruised, prop it up so that it rests above waist
level and apply a hot water bottle at a comfortably warm

temperature, which will help the blood to be absorbed back into the bloodstream more quickly.

BUMPS ON THE HEAD

A bump on the head as result of a fall can pose a danger to young and old alike. Children can easily bang their heads on the corners of tables, doors, door knobs or just from stumbling.

➕ First Aid

For mild bumps on the head you need to act quickly to minimise bruising and alleviate pain. You can do this by wringing out a clean flannel or tea towel that has been soaked in cold water and applying it to the bump. Keep doing this for about fifteen minutes, or until it feels comfortable.

For more serious bumps on the head, see Head Injuries, page 132.

BUNIONS

A painful swelling against the big toe joint is usually connected with a severely deformed joint which protrudes outwards. The bunion is caused by excessive rubbing on this protrusion.

➕ First Aid

You can protect the bunion by wearing loose-fitting shoes and by placing felt pads bought from your pharmacist over the bunion. Otherwise, consult a chiropodist.

BURNS AND SCALDS

What's the difference between a burn and a scald? The difference is quite straightforward, actually. Burns tend to be the result of skin coming into contact with a dry kind of heat, such as a flame or an electric iron, whereas scalds – in most people's minds – are caused by the skin coming into contact with wet heat, usually steam or boiling water. However, doctors don't differentiate between a scald and a 'dry' burn, because boiling water can burn the skin right through just like other forms of burn.

For chemical burns, see page 63.

✚ First Aid

✳ Minor burns

To treat minor burns or scalds, just cool the area under ordinary cold mains tap water – perhaps by keeping it running on the burned tissues for at least five or ten minutes. Then cover it with a clean, dry dressing, which cuts down the danger of infection. If you don't have a first aid dressing, a clean handkerchief or tea towel will serve as an interim measure.

Some people find that briefly rubbing the sore area with an ice cube can help – but do run water over the ice cube first to prevent the skin being damaged further by the ice sticking to it.

Remove anything tight near the burn, perhaps a ring or a watch strap, because burnt skin can swell up and any restrictions would make it even more painful or hinder circulation.

You can also soothe the sore area with creams and sprays specially made for burns and scalds. Most contain an antiseptic and some sprays contain mepyramine maleate, an antihistamine, and benzocaine, a local anaesthetic.

Burns or scalds can damage the skin and so make it liable to infection. That's why it's important never to burst a blister that might form on the burned or scalded area. By doing that you'll only let germs in rather than keeping them out.

✳ Serious burns

Even a minor burn which is bigger than a 5 cm square should be seen by a doctor. Superficial burns may hurt more than serious ones because a deeper burn may have destroyed the nerve endings, so you can no longer feel the pain. With much larger burns, the damaged – or absent – skin cannot prevent the body's water and chemicals from seeping out and evaporating. The subsequent risk of dehydration with a large burn can be a greater threat than the burn itself.

Don't take off burnt clothes which are stuck to the skin, but do take off any items of clothing that are soaked in hot fat, boiling water or chemicals, provided they're not stuck to the skin. Treat for shock (page 180) if the burn is large and the patient is obviously distressed.

With a boiling water burn, quickly put it under a running cold tap – ideally the mains tap usually found in a kitchen. Afterwards, if it covers a large area – especially on a child – cover with a clean cloth and go to the nearest Accident and Emergency department.

WARNING

Don't put butter on a burn no matter what your granny tells you. It retains heat and is not sterile, therefore carrying with it the risk of infection.

Prevention

Of course, burns are sometimes accidents that cannot be avoided. But in the home, for instance, do try to be careful, particularly when children are around. Children have been known to die after climbing into a bathful of water that was far too hot for them while Mum wasn't looking. It's a good idea to pour in cold water before adding hot.

Keep kettles or teapots away from the edges of worktops or tables. The water in such containers can scald up to half an hour after the water has boiled! A seemingly innocent cup of tea can cause very bad burns. Never drink one while holding a baby at the same time.

Turn saucepan handles away from the edges of cookers and have them pointed sideways, whether there are children around or not. You too could easily brush against the handle. Take care when you use pressure cookers – escaping steam can cause scalding. Be extra careful when using hot oil, especially chip pans, or even lifting roast potatoes out of the oven – if dropped, the fat in the roasting tray can cause nasty burns to your legs and feet even if it only splashes against you.

Always use well-padded oven gloves when you are taking something hot out of the oven. The oven door could be hot enough to burn, not just the dish inside. Be careful too when using microwaves, particularly when you are heating drinks. Make sure you stir any drink thoroughly. There could be 'heat spots' which will burn your mouth, or sometimes drinks can boil over the edges of cups after they have been in microwaves.

Always use safety fireguards in front of any fire, be it coal, electric or gas. Radiators and hot water pipes can cause burns as well, so avoid touching them and keep children away from them.

Be careful, too, when you are ironing. So many people cause minor burns to their hands or forearms while they are doing this chore. Concentrate on what you are doing, not the film on telly that you may be watching while you work. Make sure you rest the iron safely, preferably flat and not on its heel, on the iron rest of your ironing board. And whether ironing or boiling a kettle always make sure that there are no trailing flexes which can be tripped over or pulled by inquisitive children.

CAR ACCIDENTS

If you are involved in a car crash and you have escaped severe injury, you first need to check whether the other passengers are OK. Crush injuries (see page 82) may have occurred and also whiplash, when the head is forcibly bent first forwards with the impact and then backwards with the bounce back (see page 213). The severity of this may not be immediately apparent since often the muscle spasm and pain the injury causes may take time to appear.

You need to seek emergency help but make sure you don't endanger yourself or other passengers by leaving them in dangerous positions when they can't fend for themselves. If possible turn on the hazard lights.

Likewise, if you witness a road traffic accident, you need to get an ambulance first, then go over to the scene without endangering yourself. For first aid at a serious accident, see Alive or Dead?, page 10.

BE CAREFUL!

Make sure your baby or child rides in a properly secured car seat. Don't carry a baby in your arms in a car . Don't think that they will be safe if you put a safety belt around the both of you. They won't. The baby could be crushed if you were to be in a car accident.

CHEMICAL BURNS

Chemical burns differ from burns caused by flames or dry heat, such as the surface of an electric iron, in that their effects may not be evident immediately. Chemicals that burn can be found in most homes: for example, some paint strippers, acids in car batteries, even bleach.

🛇 Signs and Symptoms

At first you may notice some stinging, followed by a discoloration of the skin. The skin may also become red and very sore. There will be blistering or even peeling in some cases.

➕ First Aid

You must follow the same principles as for treating any other burn. Run tap water over the area, but with chemical burns you'll need to let the water run over the burned skin for quite a bit longer – until you are sure that all the chemical has been washed off and is no longer able to cause further harm.

✳ Chemical burns to the eye

If chemicals are inadvertently splashed into your eye you need to get to a basin or sink as quickly as you can and allow cold tap water to run over your eye for a minimum of ten minutes. Make sure your injured eye is nearest the basin so that water which could contain minute traces of the chemical doesn't splash into your good eye. Once that's done, cover the eye with a clean dressing and get yourself to hospital quickly.

Resist the temptation to rub your eye: should there be much inflammation you'll make it worse and more likely to get infected. And if the eye's window at the front – the cornea – is ulcerated, rubbing can make it worse and the subsequently larger scar may cover the line of vision after the ulcer has healed, considerably diminishing sight or making it bad enough to require a corneal transplant.

CHEST PAINS

Most people's immediate thought, if they notice a pain in their chest, is could this be a heart attack? Of course, chest pain could mean you are having a heart attack but please rest assured that there are many other causes: a specialist would list at least twenty. So the important thing if you experience any worrying attacks of chest pain is to be examined by your doctor so that he or she can make a definite diagnosis and hopefully rule out any serious disorders.

The doctor will first listen carefully to your description of the type of pain. He or she will know that people commonly use words like 'stabbing', 'pricking', 'niggling', 'stinging' and 'stitch-like' to describe pain due to problems unrelated to the heart. When heart disease is the underlying cause, words like 'crushing', 'excruciating', 'gripping', 'heavy' or 'bursting' tend to be used.

✸ Possible causes

As well as angina (see page 31) or a heart attack (see page 135), pain could be due to inflammation of the capsule surrounding the heart (pericarditis) because of an infection, or valve problems within the heart.

However, chest pain can come from many other sources – from various lung conditions, from muscle or bone problems in the rib cage or spine, from a hiatus hernia (see page 143) causing heartburn, as well as referred pain from a peptic ulcer or gall bladder disease, for example. Sometimes, attacks of angina can be due to an underlying condition such as an overactive thyroid gland which, if treated, often cures the angina. Shingles, too, can cause pains around the chest surface.

> *Intercostal cramp*
> Sometimes, simple cramp in the tiny muscles between the ribs (called intercostal cramp) can cause temporary acute pain, usually relieved by taking a deep breath.

✱ Viral infection

A viral infection (with the Coxsackie B virus) called Bornholm's disease or 'Devil's grip' can cause sudden severe pain in the chest and abdomen which can be mistaken for a heart attack. A small epidemic may develop in an area as the virus is infectious but symptoms usually subside on their own in about a week. Painkillers should relieve the pain once the diagnosis is made. Your pharmacist will advise you on a suitable product.

✱ Spontaneous pneumothorax

A spontaneous pneumothorax of a kind that causes the pressure to rise on one side of the lung's cavity can also cause sudden severe pain similar to a heart attack. A pneumothorax – due to a hole developing in the lung – causes air to leak from the lungs into the pleural cavity – the space between the lining of the chest wall and that of the lungs.

✱ Inflammation

Pleurisy, an inflammation of the lung lining due to an infection or a blockage in its blood supply, can be painful, too.

Osteochondritis, sometimes known as Tietze's disease, is another fairly common reason for sudden chest pain. An inflammation occurs at the point where a rib joins the breast-bone and the joint can be extremely tender and may be swollen. The cause is unknown. Anti-inflammatory, pain-relieving tablets, or an injection into the joint, may be recommended.

➕ First Aid

With so many possible reasons for chest pain, it is essential to consult a doctor and various investigations may be needed to get to the cause of the problem. Aspirin given to an adult (in those not sensitive to it) will both relieve pain and start a recognised treatment if a heart attack is suspected.

CHICKENPOX

Chickenpox is a common infection. It's contagious and is caused by a virus called herpes zoster. The same virus also causes shingles. More often than not chickenpox is caught in

> *What should I do?*
> Should you take your child to the doctor's surgery? It's advisable to notify your doctor that your child is covered with a rash that looks like chickenpox. Then you'll be able to discuss the best course of action with him or her.

childhood, when it's less severe than in adulthood. Once you've had it you'll be immune to it, although, having said that, the virus can lie dormant and later on in life may cause shingles.

🛈 Signs and Symptoms

Chickenpox is likely to be developing when you see a rash or crops of small red spots appearing on the body and then spreading to the arms, legs, face and head. These spots then change to watery blisters that either burst or shrivel up and crust over. The virus can make you feel generally unwell and there may be a raised temperature.

The incubation period of the virus is about seventeen days from the first contact. The rash will usually become 'quiet' in seven days, but scabs may be obvious for up to four weeks.

➕ First Aid

Calamine lotion can help to soothe the eruption. Try not to scratch as this can cause infection. Paracetamol – particularly for children – will help lower any raised temperature. A medicine may be prescribed to soothe the itching and antihistamine medicines supplied by your pharmacist can also bring relief.

> *Keep well away?*
> Do you need to keep the child away from other children? As a rule of thumb, most doctors say that the child can go to school a week after the rash first appears, providing that the child feels well enough to do so. This is because the child was most infectious in the days just before the rash came out.

CHILBLAINS

Chilblains are reddish-blue discolorations of the skin usually affecting the toes, fingers and backs of the legs. They're caused by exposure to cold, which is why you are more likely to develop them in winter. They affect more women than men and more young women than old.

What happens is that the blood flow through the body, especially to the extremities – fingers, toes and ears – is interrupted as the small blood vessels constrict in the tissues of the sufferer. This is a natural occurrence, as the body automatically supplies less blood to the skin surface in order to retain essential heat deep within the tissues (for the body to function properly, the kidneys, the heart and particularly the brain and the blood have to keep a constant temperature around the normal 37°C/98.4°F mark).

But with chilblain sufferers this natural defence mechanism causes problems. Those small vessels remain closed up tightly for longer than usual. When the fingers or toes of someone with a tendency to chilblains are exposed to warmth, the previously cold tissues come 'alive' again before their blood supply returns to normal because the small vessels don't open up quickly enough. Pain and discomfort are felt because not enough oxygen is getting to the now warm tissues which, as a result of being warm again, are in need of it.

Because of this absence of an adequate supply of oxygen the tissues become more alkaline when they are warmed, a further cause of pain and itching until the local 'chemistry' is restored to normality. When the blood vessels eventually open again the pain and numbness disappear.

🛈 Signs and Symptoms

Symptoms include burning, itching and pain in the fingers, toes, back of the legs or ears. Chilblains can be accompanied by swelling and when severe can ulcerate.

✚ First Aid

Treat chilblains by covering them with a loose, dry dressing such as gauze and, if you wish, applying a soothing antiseptic cream. A vapour rub (providing the skin is unbroken) may help increase blood flow, as the rubbing stimulates circulation.

You can put hands or feet into a bowl of lukewarm (not hot) water to revive them. Having a warm drink, such as a cup of tea, will help warm you too. Don't use a hot water bottle and it's probably wise not to use one in bed at night if you suffer from chilblains for the reasons given under 'Be Careful!' below.

When you get chilblains for the first time, or if they are severe, consult your doctor in order to rule out any more serious problems such as Raynaud's phenomenon or even Lupus Erythematosis. (Although causes are not known precisely, Raynaud's symptoms are due to the blood vessels becoming over-sensitive – especially to the effects of cold. Lupus Erythematosis is an auto-immune condition in which the body's defences 'attack' its own tissues.)

If you are prone to chilblains, keep hands and feet warm in cold weather.

BE CAREFUL!

If your hands and feet become very cold, don't subject them to immediate warmth. They need to be warmed up slowly. Trying to rush the process can harm the tissues and cause lots more pain.

CHIPPED BONES

See Broken Bones, page 55.

CHOKING

Anyone choking on food needs help, be they young or old. Don't just sit there. Do something!

BE CAREFUL!
Don't waste time trying to grab hold of the constricting object with your fingers, unless it is obvious and easy to pick out. If it's not obvious you could cause further harm by pushing it back into the windpipe.

✚ First Aid

✳ Choking in an adult

You need to hold the person firmly below the lower chest and jerk inwards with your interlocked hands to thrust air out of the lung to dislodge the obstruction. Repeat again up to four times. You do this by standing behind the victim. Push one of your fists with thumb inward against the stomach. Interlock your fist with your other fist in order to thrust inwards and upwards under the rib cage.

Or you can sit the person on a chair, making them lean forwards. Use the flat of your hand to slap the victim between the shoulder blades several times.

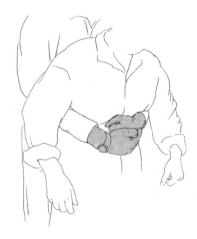

✳ Choking in a baby

Hold the baby upside down, supporting him on the inside of your forearm. As a guide, his bottom should lie in the crease of your elbow and your open hand should support his chest.

Slap the baby's back smartly between the shoulder blades. If the object doesn't come out, do it again. If after several attempts you still haven't dislodged whatever is causing the obstruction, give the baby's tummy a short quick squeeze. This should push the object out of the baby's windpipe.

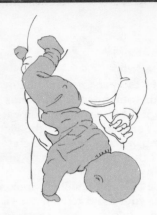

✳ Choking in a child

For a child over the age of nine years deal as with an adult but use only one fist and not quite as much force.

For a child under nine years, you can quickly put them over your lap with the face pointing downwards. The head should be angled below your knees. Give several sharp slaps between the shoulder blades.

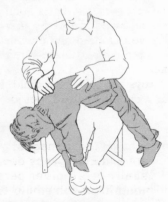

✳ When you're on your own

Quickly grab a chair or use the edge of a worktop. Lean over the back of the chair and hold on with the hands placed at each side. Then thrust inwards and upwards just below your ribcage three or four times. This will help to force air out of your lungs to dislodge the obstruction.

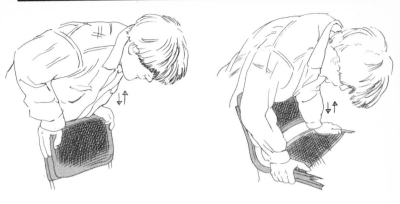

Prevention

For future reference, don't give peanuts to a child under the age of five. You may think that they can manage them, but they do pose a choking hazard. In addition, the oil in the nut can cause swelling if a fragment becomes trapped, which can in turn lead to an attack of pneumonia. Be careful about giving a baby or toddler hard foods which may be a little too much for them to deal with. Boiled sweets aren't a good idea. Raw apple or raw carrot should be avoided for the first two years. And never leave a baby or young child alone while they are eating. Also check bottle teats regularly to make sure they aren't beginning to wear or break.

Think about the toys you give your child. Even a soft cuddly toy could provide a choking hazard, not just from its eyes or

For food stuck in the gullet (oesophagus) get the person to a hospital Accident and Emergency department without delay. It will usually be an older person who has swallowed a large mouthful of something quite solid, for example a partially chewed piece of meat. They will be quite distressed and may feel a constricting tightness in their chest. They will usually complain that something's got stuck in their throat. The spasm of the gullet may also be causing considerable pain, adding to their distress.

nose, which could become dislodged and then swallowed, but from the pile fabric or monofilament used to simulate fur or hair – these fabrics are a hazard particularly for young children who tend to put things in their mouths.

And when you're eating, do just that – eat – don't do something else at the same time.

COLD SORES

Cold sores are caused by the herpes simplex type I virus – one of the herpes group of viruses. (Others in this group cause chickenpox, shingles and glandular fever.) It's a common virus which is around most of the time.

Signs and Symptoms

The first symptoms of cold sores are pain and tingling sensations usually around the lips, although cold sores can appear on other parts of the body.

Cold sores are little blisters which develop into weeping sores. They usually appear in groups around the lips but may also occur on other parts of the face. If the blisters break, the wound will be swarming with the virus germs, which can easily be passed on to someone else by touching or kissing.

First Aid

First aid for cold sores is now better than ever, since you can buy an excellent anti-viral treatment from your pharmacist. And if Zovirax, an anti-viral cream, is applied at the first sign of trouble, it may quell the infection so the germs don't nest in the cells. It's also useful in subsequent outbreaks if used when warning symptoms occur before the sores appear – that 'prickly' feeling in the area of skin usually affected – because it can shorten the duration of the outbreak considerably. But if the virus nests, it is inclined to break out again whenever the body's defences are run down as a result of a cold (hence the name) or other illness. The pain of outbreaks can be relieved by painkillers, or by a cream such as Blisteze.

If you don't have any creams at hand, you can use fresh,

> *Did you know?*
> The cold sore virus cannot be passed on while it is dormant and producing no symptoms. But when you are infectious it is essential to protect others.

cold coffee dabbed on the area with a piece of clean cotton wool every two or three hours. It may sound primitive, but it appears to work for many people, so it is worth trying if a doctor or pharmacist isn't available. Other than this, the sores should just be kept clean and dry.

✳ Containing the outbreak

You can infect vulnerable parts of your own body, via the fingers, if you touch the sores and do not wash your hands afterwards. Any area of broken skin is especially susceptible. It is particularly important to avoid touching the blisters and then rubbing the eyes, as the virus may be transferred and cause an ulcer on the delicate membrane covering the eye. If this is not diagnosed and treated soon enough, it can damage the sight.

Mothers with cold sores should take extra care and wash their hands frequently, and always after applying cold-sore medication. Babies and toddlers are extremely vulnerable to cold sores as they won't have had time to build up their antibodies. It is also important to keep the flannels, towels and eating and drinking utensils of the sufferer separate from those of the rest of the family.

COLDS

The common cold is a virus infection that is spread from one person to another by droplet infection – the usually unseen aerosol of droplets blown into the air when someone with a cold breathes out and especially when they cough or sneeze.

The cold viruses 'going around' tend to change constantly and none of them can be 'cured' by medicines. They can be fought and destroyed only by your body's natural defences. So those of us who mix with people regularly can expect to meet and succumb to two or three colds a year. But do remember that a cold tends to go of its own accord in a few days!

❗ Signs and Symptoms

* an unpleasant tingling sensation in the nose and throat
* sneezing
* coughing
* a temperature in the worst cases – though usually only raised by a degree or so

➕ First Aid

First aid for colds means taking aspirin or paracetamol in an adult and paracetamol in a child to relieve the worst of the symptoms and help to bring any raised temperature back to normal. (Beware of cold remedies which contain paracetamol. Don't take more than the maximum daily dose of paracetamol.) Drink plenty of fluids, too. Inhaling 'steam' coming off a bowl of very hot water – with added recommended inhalants from the pharmacy if you wish – can soothe and relieve nasal, throat or bronchial congestion.

Tepid sponging may cool and soothe children. As long as they have plenty of liquids, don't worry too much if they refuse to eat – their appetites recover very quickly. But do call your doctor if your child develops a high fever, persistent coughing, wheezing, earache or sickness.

Did you know?
About a hundred different viruses have been shown to cause the symptoms of a cold. This is one of the reasons why we continue to catch them, since even if we build up our antibodies to the cold germ that we've just had, another can come along and immediately take hold should we breathe in a sufficiently large number of germs from another sufferer. Also, the antibodies that we do produce are short lived. Consequently, the same virus can cause another cold very shortly afterwards if we are re-infected with it.

COLIC

Colic in babies is caused by bubbles of gas or air which become trapped in the immature digestive system. Problems with colic often appear when the baby is about three weeks old. They can be very wearing for the parents as well as the child, but don't despair, they usually stop of their own accord at about three months.

If a doctor's examination, repeated several times, fails to uncover any cause for crying, yet the baby continues to thrive, put on weight and develop normally, then colic is usually the diagnosis.

❗ Signs and Symptoms

The pain of colic makes the baby cry, often inconsolably, and draw his or her legs up in pain. Most parents usually learn very quickly to distinguish their baby's colic cry from a cry that means something else is wrong – such as the baby is too hot or cold, needs a nappy change or feeding, or is in pain from an injury.

➕ First Aid

There are ways you can soothe your colicky baby. Rocking or cuddling should help, and a car journey or pram ride will often send the baby off to sleep.

Giving the age-old but new-formulated remedy of gripe water can help relieve the colicky pains, wind and troublesome hiccups. Another type of medicine, such as Infacol, which is a sugar-free, alcohol-free and colorant-free liquid, will help relieve infant colic and griping pain and also effectively assist in bringing up wind. It contains activated dimethicone, which helps any trapped gas bubbles join to form bigger bubbles which the baby can bring up easily. It's suitable for babies of all ages. It has a build-up effect which means it should be given for several days to achieve the best results.

Make sure you give your baby lots of love, and wind him or her regularly until the phase passes. But always ask your health visitor or doctor for advice the first time your baby screams inconsolably. And once your doctor has told you your baby

> *Crying and babies*
> I'm sometimes asked about babies crying so long and hard that they go blue in the face. Many babies, indeed children, can work themselves up into such a frenzy their throat muscles go into a spasm. Fortunately, though, these muscles will eventually relax of their own accord and the child should get back to breathing normally again.
>
> However, it's always wise to seek the advice of your doctor or health visitor, just to check your child has nothing medically wrong.

suffers from colic, don't be frightened to ask for advice again if there are any sudden changes or worsening in the symptoms. You can only let worry be your guide when you are not medically trained.

COMAS

Coma refers to the state in which a casualty is unconscious and cannot be roused, even when pinched.

See also Alive or Dead?, page 10.

CONCUSSION

If someone is knocked unconscious for a short time following a head blow, they could be concussed. Concussion occurs when the brain is shaken. This can happen because it is 'floating' in a liquid – the cerebro-spinal fluid – and is attached to the inside of the skull by ligaments. This protects its delicate structures from many slight knocks, which are absorbed by the liquid. But with a larger knock, the brain gets bumped from side to side and may get 'bruised' as a result.

🛈 Signs and Symptoms

Anyone who suffers a head injury that causes a loss of consciousness can be considered to be concussed.

Concussion can occur after all head injuries of any severity. There doesn't have to be an open wound or fracture.

Someone who appears to be mentally confused, either immediately after the injury or in the twenty-four hours or so that follow is likely to be concussed. The worry is that some of the brain's vital functions – unconsciously controlling the body's blood pressure, normal temperature and oxygen levels, for example – will be affected, threatening the person's life.

➕ First Aid

To be on the safe side, therefore, someone who has been knocked unconscious will need to be checked every fifteen minutes for twenty-four hours after the accident to make sure everything is working properly. This is usually achieved by admitting them to hospital so that regular bedside checks can be made.

If following a head injury the sufferer appears confused, with or without a headache, lie them down, in the recovery position if they find it comfortable (see page 18), and call for professional help.

COT DEATH

A 'cot death' is when a baby is found dead in its cot without any warning: that is, when there had been no signs that they were suffering from any illness. And most often there are no traces of illness even after the event.

It is important to remember that cot death, while being the most frequent cause of death in babies up to the age of one year, is still very rare. So please do get the problem into perspective and don't worry needlessly. That's why I feel it deserves a mention here, not just because you'll need to know what to do in the case of such an emergency, but also because of the extent of worry it causes parents.

According to the Foundation for the Study of Infant Deaths, in 1991 1134 babies under one year died as a result of cot deaths in the UK. In 1992, following a campaign to reduce these statistics, the number of deaths dropped to 613, for which the campaign must take some credit.

> *Try to revive*
> If you find your baby unconscious in his or her cot or pram, always start resuscitation procedures immediately (see Mouth-to-Mouth Resuscitation, page 16). Send for help and continue until otherwise advised. Even if the baby appears to be lifeless, not breathing and without a pulse, this may have only recently occurred and revival procedures could still be life saving.

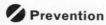 **Prevention**

Guidelines for reducing the risk of cot death are what they say they are – guidelines. There is no advice which can guarantee the prevention of cot death. As recommended by the FSID, they are:

* Place your baby on his or her back or side to sleep.
* Don't smoke and avoid smoky atmospheres.
* Do not let your baby get too hot.
* If you think your baby is unwell, contact your doctor.

Sleeping on the back or, if your baby prefers, on the side is best because there is a very marginal link between babies sleeping on their tummies and some cot deaths. It is thought that the connection could be to do with overheating. Don't let your baby get too hot even if he or she is unwell.

Smoking has been shown to increase the risk of cot death. Mothers who smoke during pregnancy tend to have babies with a low birth weight, a factor linked to cot death. Low birth weight can also be shown, on average, to be associated with most health problems that can befall a baby, although the majority will be fine. It is a statistical risk. But since smoking can be avoided, why add to your baby's risks by smoking, or allowing smoking in your presence or that of the baby?

But even when parents have followed all these guidelines and reduced the risks overall, there will still be some babies who suffer a cot death because we don't always know precisely why cot deaths occur. And when they do, usually without any obvious explanation, even the very best of parents will blame themselves and ask where they went wrong. The answer is: they didn't.

COUGHING UP BLOOD

Coughing up blood must always be considered to be due to a potentially serious disease until proven otherwise. It is essential – and may be vital – to seek your doctor's advice without delay.

It is also important to determine whether the blood has been coughed up or vomited up, as this will obviously help the doctor's diagnosis (see page 45). Treat for shock (page 180), if necessary.

COUGHS

Coughing is a natural response to any foreign body, congestion or irritation in the lungs or throat. It's not an illness in itself, but a symptom of, for example, irritation from air pollution or cigarette smoke, or the result of an infection.

Signs and Symptoms

Coughs can occur as a consequence of the common cold or flu. These often sound chesty and you may cough up phlegm.

A cough can also be dry. This type occurs when there is irritation but little phlegm in the larynx at the top of the wind pipe, or in the pharynx, the cavern between the mouth and nose at the top, and the oesophagus (gullet) and trachea (wind pipe) below. This irritation stimulates the cough reflex – the body's natural response.

First Aid

Cough medicines can relieve the irritation or embarrassment of a cough. There are many types available and it is wise to ask your pharmacist to suggest the type of remedy most suitable for your particular problem. In the main, though, expectorants are said to relieve chesty coughs as they loosen the 'debris' or phlegm so it is easier to cough up. Others contain cough suppressants to halt the symptoms. They reduce the frequency and intensity of a cough by acting on the part of the brain that controls the coughing reflex, or at the site of irritation in the throat. Other medicines contain decongestants to help clear nasal pasages or soothing substances such as honey and glycerine to act on the throat's surface – in fact if you don't have any cough medicine and are unable to get to a pharmacy, a drink of honey, lemon juice and warm water may be soothing.

> ### BE CAREFUL!
>
> Sometimes, however, coughing signals a more serious disorder in the respiratory tract. So it is extremely important to seek medical advice for any cough that lasts for longer than a few days or if there are streaks of blood in any mucus you cough up. Coughing up green sputum probably signifies a bacterial infection and you'll need to seek your doctor's advice.

CRAMP

Cramp is a sudden, violent muscle contraction which makes the muscle become hard and tense. It is usually caused by exercise, especially unaccustomed exercise, or a prolonged period of sitting, lying or standing in an awkward position. No one really knows what causes it. It may occasionally be the result of poor blood supply due to the furring up of the arteries – this is especially likely with elderly sufferers. Some drugs – diuretics, for example – can also make cramp more likely by altering the body's chemical balance. Occasionally an underlying condition, such as a thyroid or nerve disorder, can cause muscular cramps, so do consult your doctor if it persists. (See also Intercostal Cramp, page 64.)

🛈 Signs and Symptoms

A sudden, painful muscle spasm, most often in the calf, thigh or foot (though it can develop anywhere). The spasm can be very painful.

> *Each to his own*
> Many people swear by having a string of corks under their pillow at night. Others put potatoes in their beds, or magnets under their mattress. As far as I know, there's no scientific evidence that these 'cures' work, but if they seem to help you, and are harmless, that's good enough reason to use them!

➕ First Aid

With the most common sort of cramp, in the calf muscles, try this:

1 Stand facing a wall and at arm's length from it.
2 Place the flat of your hands against the wall and slowly bend forward from the ankles so that your calves are gently but comfortably stretched.
3 Do this standing 'press-up' six times on three separate occasions throughout the day and continue it for ten days.

This exercise will also flex the ankles and stretch the soles of the feet because another common site for cramp is in the instep of the foot which often wakes sufferers in the night.

Massaging and stretching the cramped muscle, immersing it in hot water, or warming it with a hot water bottle may also bring relief.

CROUP

Croup is an infection of the throat and windpipe which can cause swelling, and in young children can become a medical emergency.

❗ Signs and Symptoms

Symptoms are likely to be a high temperature with noisy coughing and breathing as well as a hoarse voice.

First Aid

The distress of croup is due to congestion of the bronchial tubes which can occur when an infection is present. Any breathing difficulties of this nature should be referred to your doctor because the child may need antibiotics. A child's tubes are small in diameter, and infection can easily constrict the passage of air. The dry air being breathed in makes a rasping noise as it grates down the narrow tubes, so it's necessary to moisten the air in order to lubricate its flow.

The quickest way to increase moisture in the air is to boil a kettle. Leave a kettle boiling for a minute in your child's room, then switch it off and remove the lid. The kettle will continue to give off water vapour even though you may not be able to see the steam.

An alternative is to run a small amount of hot water into the bath, then wrap your child up well and take him or her into the bathroom. The water will moisten the air and his breathing will ease in moments.

If there is a harsh, high-pitched sound – called stridor by doctors – the sufferer will usually be very distressed since there is then a severe restriction in breathing. This can be caused by inflammation of the epiglottis – epiglottitis – which can occur in both adults and children. A sufferer needs to be taken to an Accident and Emergency department without delay. If in doubt, phone your doctor immediately.

CRUSH INJURIES

This type of injury must always be treated as serious, and medical help must be sought immediately. Crush injuries – the type cyclists suffer as a result of being run over by a car, for example – can damage areas of the body badly. They can happen at home, too, for instance when children are playing in a bedroom and pull a wardrobe down on top of them. The worst one I've ever seen was when a workman, working at the bottom of a lift shaft, had the lift descend on him, squeezing him into the space at the bottom.

> *Tourniquets and the Crush Syndrome*
> Even tourniquets (see page 23) applied for too long can cause the Crush Syndrome. This occurs because the muscle swells after the tourniquet has been left on for too long and is then released. The nearly moribund and now swelling muscle is restricted or crushed by its own sheath and can cause the effects described below. Yet another reason for avoiding the use of a tourniquet.

🛈 Signs and Symptoms

Tissues, such as muscles, can be damaged, bones can be fractured, there can be swelling and there is the risk of 'Crush Syndrome'. This is due to the waste products from a crushed muscle clogging up the kidneys, preventing them from functioning properly. Consequently other waste products, normally cleared from the body by the kidneys, start to build up. The urine output falls over the next few days, the patient becomes apathetic and restless and may even become delirious.

During crush injuries, the chest may be damaged, making unaided breathing difficult. Internal organs may also be crushed, leading to internal bleeding and shock.

✚ First Aid

Call for help and, without moving the individual if this is possible, remove the cause of the crush. Take measures to sustain life until professional help arrives.

The Crush Syndrome requires treatment in hospital with careful management of the person's liquid intake among other measures.

The crushed muscle will often swell within its tough and unyielding covering sheath. This may need to be cut in places to relieve the pressure building up and so prevent further crushing of the muscle.

CUTS AND LACERATIONS

You can treat most cuts and lacerations at home quite safely, but always wash your hands first, if possible.

❗ Signs and Symptoms

A break in the skin with mild to minor bleeding.

➕ First Aid

✳ Cleaning the cut

Allowing the cut to bleed freely for a few seconds is helpful because this is nature's way of flushing out dirt and germs. Additionally, clean the cut by holding it under running water, or by gently wiping it with an antiseptic wipe or piece of cotton wool soaked in warm water.

It is best to use a fresh piece of cotton wool for each wipe. Some small cuts will bleed quite profusely at first but most will usually stop of their own accord after a little while.

✳ Stopping the bleeding

Bleeding in a normal person will stop in time when pressure is applied. When it doesn't it could imply that there is a foreign body present, or the blood clotting mechanism is faulty. If the bleeding continues after a few minutes, you'll need to apply pressure to stem the flow. Press a pad, a clean tissue for example, firmly over the cut for a few minutes. Some bleeding can take as long as ten minutes or so to stop.

If it is a cut on the leg or arm you could also raise the limb, because this, together with the applied pressure, will help to stop bleeding. But don't do this if the cut appears to be accompanied by a fracture.

✳ Dressings

Large wounds will need to have the edges pressed together. Use both hands to do this, before applying a dressing, as shown in the diagram.

If you like to use plasters and antiseptic ointments on cuts and grazes, fine – they will do no harm. Personally, I prefer not

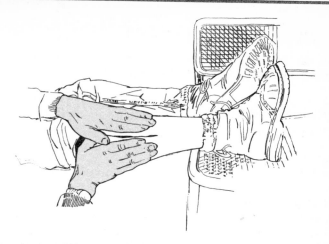

to use ointments and I use plasters mainly to keep dirt out of the wound. When that isn't necessary or the injury is small, it will heal up nicely if left alone.

✳ Cuts from broken glass

Broken glass can be just as sharp as a knife wound and can produce nasty cuts. Very often, for example, innocent by-standers suffer severe injuries from broken glass as a result of a terrorist bomb explosion. The other problem posed by cuts from glass is that the glass can shatter into tiny splinters that are difficult to see. If you think that glass splinters may be in a wound, take the person to a hospital Accident and Emergency department and let the professionals sort it out.

Always be aware of the dangers of glass, particularly if you have children around. It's a good idea to keep glasses, glass ornaments and bowls away from inquisitive young hands.

✳ Cuts doing DIY

A large percentage of cuts are caused by people doing DIY, particularly when using a knife or a saw. Clean the cut by running under water and follow the general advice for cuts shown above. If the cut is deep or wide you will possibly need stitches. While such cuts do not usually pose a risk of tetanus, they often provide an opportunity to see that your tetanus injections are up to date so make sure you check this (see page 22).

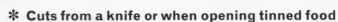

✽ Cuts from a knife or when opening tinned food

For dealing with knife cuts during food preparation or when opening tins, follow the instructions for cuts in general. Make certain that if a cut is longer than one centimetre or quite deep your doctor or practice nurse checks it out.

Take special care when opening corned beef tins which are frequently irregularly shaped. Children can easily cut their fingers on the tops of canned drinks, so watch them carefully.

✽ Paper cuts

If you cut yourself on the edge of a piece of paper, just run your finger under water. If the cut bleeds for more than a few minutes, press hard with a clean cloth. Small cuts of this nature heal quickly when left uncovered.

✽ Shaving cuts

Cutting yourself while shaving has the advantage of being clean and anyway, since the advent of safety razors, shaving 'injuries' have been more nicks than cuts. To stop the bleeding, try pressing the cut with a clean flannel. If that works there will be little surrounding blood left to look unsightly. If, as is more usual, it won't because the moisture is not allowing the blood to clot, use a small piece of clean cotton wool and press with your finger until the bleeding stops.

Remove any excess cotton wool leaving the last small piece in place to provide extra clot support – and a point of interest for many people throughout the day!

Women frequently cut their legs when shaving them and such cuts, though minor, can produce quite a lot of blood.

✽ Cutting your tongue

As with a nose bleed, when we cut our tongue it often appears that the injury is more serious than it really is because

---

Did you know?
When stitches are put into a wound, the wound heals by second intention, not from the bottom up, but from side to side. Stitches allow the wound to heal more quickly with the result that the scar is likely to be thinner.

of the seemingly plentiful amounts of blood produced. So your first step in dealing with a cut on the tongue is don't panic. Apply pressure to the spot for a few minutes. If in doubt, seek medical help.

✽ Medical help for cuts

If any cut is very large or deep, if it has ragged or gaping edges, if something is embedded in it or if it is a deep cut with only a small opening in the skin, always seek advice. If a wound has something embedded in it, you can try to stem the flow of blood by pressing on either side of the object, keeping the injured limb or body area raised. Don't remove the object unless you can do so very easily. Cover with a dressing and get the person to hospital as quickly as you can or call for an ambulance, depending on the severity and the circumstances.

Gaping wounds or deep cuts may require stitches. A doctor will decide to put in stitches when the hole is so far apart it will heal by first intention, that is to say it heals from the bottom up. Healing this way takes longer and has the additional risk of allowing germs in to cause infection. It may also leave a bigger scar.

CYSTITIS

Cystitis is an inflammation of the bladder lining and the urethra – the tube down which urine is passed out from the bladder. It is one of the most common complaints suffered by women, and estimates suggest that more than half the women in the UK contract cystitis at some time (and it occasionally afflicts men and children too).

ⓘ Signs and Symptoms

A woman's anatomy makes her particularly prone to cystitis. Unlike a man's, her urethra is very short and the normally harmless germs around the anus are easily able to track upwards to the bladder, whose natural defences may be unable to cope with them. Some people say they suffer more from cystitis when they are 'run down'. It is likely that they feel run down because there is a niggling infection there which doesn't cause local symptoms all the time, but makes the sufferer feel under par. From time to time, however, the local symptoms will present themselves.

These symptoms could be frequent, painful urination, and the urine can also be cloudy, blood-stained and strong-smelling.

➕ First Aid

If symptoms do develop, neutralising the acidity is a worthwhile first line of treatment, since as many as two out of three sufferers won't actually have any infection. Using this method alone the symptoms should settle in a day or so if no infection is present.

Immediately symptoms appear start by drinking a pint of water with a teaspoonful of bicarbonate of soda added – unless you suffer from high blood pressure, or heart or kidney trouble, in which case consult your doctor first. Drink a pint of this mixture every hour for three hours, interspersed with other soft drinks. This will change the urine from acid to alkaline and relieve the pain, but it is not something I would recommend too often, as an excess of bicarbonate of soda, especially in a sufferer whose kidneys are not working properly, could lead to side-effects such as a rise in blood pressure.

Soluble aspirin or paracetamol can help relieve any pain in the lower abdomen, and you could ask your pharmacist about the over-the-counter products available for treating cystitis. If symptoms persist for more than two days, your doctor may prescribe antibiotics.

🚫 Prevention

Cystitis isn't always caused by an infection. The delicate lining of the urethra and/or the bladder can, in those susceptible, react to irritants such as scented soaps, powders, vaginal deodorants, bath oils and the detergents used to wash clothes. Some people are sensitive to highly spiced foods, strong tea, coffee, alcohol and fruit juices. Friction or bruising during love-making can also inflame the tissues, as the urethra is just above the vagina. A lubricant jelly may then be a good idea during intercourse to help overcome any dryness.

DEATH

In normal circumstances, if you discover someone has died, it will usually be a sick or very elderly friend or relative whom you may be caring for.

From the practical point of view, all you need do is notify their doctor. If he or she has seen them within the previous two weeks the GP will be able to issue a death certificate. If he hasn't seen them for a while, perhaps because they haven't been particularly ill recently, he will have a word with the coroner, describing the circumstances of the death and seek his advice before issuing a certificate.

If there are unusual circumstances – if the person is of no great age, there had been no previous illness and the death was totally unexpected – the coroner may order a post mortem examination to be carried out before a death certificate can be issued.

DEHYDRATION

When your body's water level drops to dangerous levels, dehydration can occur. Dehydration can be accompanied by salt depletion and can lead to headaches, lethargy, cramps and a very pale appearance. This can happen due to heat alone in the tropics. At home, the main cause is a particularly bad or prolonged attack of diarrhoea and vomiting – especially vomiting.

In a healthy person, water is essential to maintain normal body functions. Its importance is underlined by the fact that around half our body weight is water. Normally our kidneys balance the water lost in the urine and through perspiration against our fluid intake – we feel more thirsty and therefore drink more in hot weather, for instance.

🛈 Signs and Symptoms

Symptoms can include dry lips and tongue, severe thirst, your heart may beat more quickly, you can feel dizzy. In severe cases you can fall into a coma. Dehydration can mean that the body's essential minerals are lost. Mineral depletion can make you feel weak and eventually faint.

➕ First Aid

You need to seek a doctor's advice but in the meantime slowly sip water with powders added which can be bought from a pharmacy. The ready-prepared sachets are a combination of essential salts (minerals) and energy-giving glucose. This is known as oral rehydration therapy. When these are mixed with the correct quantity of water as instructed, they are just the right strength for quick absorption.

✳ DIY rehydration mixture

If you can't get to a pharmacy or contact your doctor, this is the next best thing. Mix half a level teaspoon of salt and four level teaspoons of sugar with one litre of boiled water.

This mixture is recommended by the World Health Organisation for use especially in the developing parts of the world where dehydration due to diarrhoea and vomiting can be extremely dangerous and where there is frequently no alternative either in the way of a doctor's advice or money for any medicine.

If you can manage to keep some of this down until you can get further advice, or until you can keep ordinary water and eventually bland foods down, it should help.

WARNING

If the dehydration sufferer is very young (up to four) or very old, the harmful effects of dehydration can take hold extremely quickly, so don't waste time. Seek professional medical help sooner rather than later.

DELIVERING A BABY

A first-time labour on average lasts about eighteen hours, but just as with anything else in life there are exceptions to every rule. Even in this day and age babies are born in taxis, on planes, in public toilets and even hospital car parks! And there are women who give birth without even knowing they are pregnant. So this category is worth more of a read than you first might think.

❗ Signs and Symptoms

You need to know that labour is made up of three stages.

1 The first stage is when the womb muscles begin to contract in order to open up the cervix, the neck of the womb. This stage is likely to take on average ten to twelve hours for a first baby.
2 The second stage is a much quicker process. The cervix will now have dilated fully – to a width of 10 cm – and the mother will want to begin pushing the baby out.
3 The third stage is when the placenta or afterbirth is delivered.

✳ Warning signs of imminent labour

Warning signs that a woman is going into labour are usually obvious – but having said that, some women just complain of a little backache!

* There may be a 'show', which is a plug of very thick, blood-stained jelly-like mucus. This plug seals the neck of the womb throughout pregnancy but may come away as the cervix begins to dilate.
* The woman's waters may break. This is the amniotic fluid that surrounds the baby in the womb. This could take the form of a warm trickle or for some women can involve copious amounts of fluid leaving the body with a sudden rush. Once the waters are broken it's not advisable for a woman to have a bath or shower as there is a risk of infection.
* Contractions start off as a mild backache which build up in intensity to cramping pains described as similar to bad period pains. If, in no time at all, the pains start to come very closely together, and the woman gets an uncontrollable desire to push all the time, the birth may be imminent and an emergency delivery may be required. Fortunately, this is not too common and there is usually plenty of time to be taken to the chosen place of delivery, or to get to bed, if it is to be at home, and to notify the midwife.

But if you suspect a woman is going into labour contact their midwife or doctor immediately and if urgency requires ring for an ambulance as well.

➕ First Aid

Try not to panic – easier said than done I know. But you have to deal with the situation, you can't delay childbirth. If it's going to happen, it will. Ideally you will need to scrub your hands, paying particular attention to fingernails. If you are in a public place, then you probably won't be able to do so. You may want to ask people nearby to stand around you to allow the mother some privacy – although from experience I would say that by the time a woman has got to this stage, she's oblivious to things going on around her.

Allow the mother to take up the position she feels most comfortable in.

As a general rule once you see the baby's head emerging the body will appear quite quickly. If you feel up to doing so, as the head is born, it is as well to feel that the umbilical cord is not hooked around the baby's neck. If it is, a gentle pull upon it with a hooked finger will enable you to flip it over the head or shoulder. Not to do so can delay the delivery at this critical stage when the cord is being squeezed, preventing blood passing through it. Wipe the baby's mouth clean of blood or mucus and wrap in a towel, or whatever is clean and available, to keep him or her warm until help arrives. Then hand the baby over to the mother.

BE CAREFUL!

You shouldn't smack the baby once it's delivered. It will normally start to breathe on its own and the smack administered in previous times is not considered to make any difference. And if, as some consider, the baby has an unconscious memory of those times, it could also be responsible for some future behavioural difficulties. So why do it?

And don't attempt to cut the umbilical cord yourself. That will be done either when a midwife arrives or when the mother and baby reach hospital.

❋ Soon after birth

Shortly after the child is born, the uterus will begin to contract again, this time to expel the placenta, also called the afterbirth. Hopefully by this time a midwife should have arrived, but if she hasn't you'll need to keep the placenta for her to examine.

The only unexpected and unusual delivery that I have experienced caused considerable anxiety to a taxi driver. It occurred when I was a medical student. A mother arrived at the small maternity hospital to which I had been attached for a month's practical tuition.

I was going back to my quarters in the middle of the night after attending a routine delivery. As I was approaching the unstaffed front entrance to the hospital, a woman was waddling in – legs apart, in great distress and about to collapse – accompanied by an ashen-faced taxi driver. I caught her, barged my way into the adjacent porter's office, shouting for the night sister and sending the taxi driver to fetch her in case she hadn't heard me.

I put my charge on the rug on the floor and delivered a healthy baby boy as the night sister and taxi driver arrived no more than two minutes later.

The much relieved new mother said she'd call him Michael!

DENTAL PAIN – TOOTHACHE

As well as decay, toothache can be caused by such things as a cracked filling or fractured tooth, even an abscess. Sometimes wisdom teeth can be a cause of dental pain. Our full set of adult teeth numbers thirty-two, with wisdom teeth at the very back.

Wisdom teeth appear, if they're going to, usually between the ages of eighteen and twenty-five. If they don't come through, you can forget them. However, if they get impacted – that is, if they grow irregularly, perhaps pushing into the tooth in front or distorting the line of the teeth – then a dentist will suggest removal. Depending on how difficult this is likely to be, the dentist will either take the teeth out himself or will refer the patient to a specialist.

❗ Signs and Symptoms

Pain felt deep in the gums, particularly a throbbing pain or pain stemming from a tooth when eating or drinking. In fact, any type of pain in a tooth or in the gums should always be checked out by a dentist to determine the cause and appropriate treatment.

➕ First Aid

Aspirin, paracetamol (especially for children) and ibuprofen can all be effective in treating dental pain if you have to wait for an appointment. Oil of cloves applied to the aching tooth by means of a soaked piece of cotton wool is remarkably effective at numbing the pain.

⊘ Prevention

To help prevent further attacks of toothache, brush your teeth regularly. Ideally brush them for at least three minutes after breakfast and at bedtime. The use of dental floss is recommended to remove plaque. Plaque, a thin, colourless, sticky

---

Replacing a lost tooth through injury

Can teeth be saved once they have fallen out? Yes, they can. The important thing is to act quickly. If a tooth is put back in its socket within thirty minutes it has the best chance but even if it is replaced within two hours it may well stay put for life.

The tooth must not be allowed to get dry so do not wrap it in anything. Do not scrub it or place it in disinfectant either. If it is dirty, rinse it in milk or lukewarm water, then gently try to push it back into its socket, holding it by its crown – the part usually visible in the mouth. Bite on a handkerchief to hold the tooth in place and go straight to a dentist or hospital casualty department. If you cannot replant the tooth, put it in a cup of milk, or in the mouth between teeth and cheek, to keep it moist and get to a dentist or hospital quickly!

substance, composed mainly of bacteria, is the main cause of gum problems and tooth decay as it forms almost continuously around the teeth and gum margins. If not removed by regular brushing and flossing it can build up and harden into a deposit known as tartar or calculus, which attracts further plaque. Tartar, unlike plaque, can be felt with the tongue and can only be removed by a dentist or dental hygienist using special instruments to scale the teeth.

* Milk teeth

When a child's milk tooth has dropped out, you'll need to press the area with a clean cloth to stop any bleeding. (See also Teething, page 208.)

DIABETES

More than a million people suffer from diabetes in the UK. A recent report in the *British Medical Journal* points out that the incidence of diabetes in children under fifteen has nearly doubled over the last fifteen years. Diabetes is a condition in which the body can't properly use sugar and carbohydrates from the food eaten. It's insulin that enables body tissues to take up glucose from the blood. The cause of diabetes is the failure of the pancreas to produce insulin and the reason why this happens is still being investigated. In children, viruses have been suggested to play a part but I believe it's down to our genes – at least in part.

There are two types of diabetes:

1 Insulin-dependent diabetes is treated by insulin injections and diet. About one in four people with diabetes have this type. It is the most severe form and usually develops under the age of thirty.
2 Non-insulin dependent diabetes affects the remaining three out of four people with diabetes. It's also known as maturity-onset diabetes and is more common among elderly people, particularly those who are overweight. With this type of diabetes insulin is produced, but not in the amounts the body needs.

Warning signs of diabetes can include feeling very thirsty, eating and drinking more, tiredness and a frequent need to pass urine. Non-insulin dependent diabetes is treated by diet alone (a reduction in the consumption of calories, especially sugary foods), or, for about half of the people with this form of diabetes, with drugs and diet. The drugs stimulate extra insulin production.

Losing weight and taking more exercise may be all that's needed for some people to control their non-insulin dependent diabetes.

✳ Diabetic emergencies

There are two types of diabetic coma:

1 Hyper-glycaemic coma comes on slowly over a matter of days as the sugar concentration builds up in the blood.
2 Hypo-glycaemic coma is when the sugar content in the blood falls dramatically and dangerously. Such hypo-glycaemia can happen in a matter of minutes to an hour.

❗ Signs and Symptoms

When a diabetic coma is mentioned the problem is usually a hyper-glycaemic coma. It is, regrettably, often the first sign that an individual has diabetes. It can occur later, after diagnosis, if the sufferer allows the diabetes to get out of control – doesn't take their insulin, for example.

Hypo-glycaemic coma usually occurs to a known sufferer when they've had to take more exercise than they were expecting, and they had not eaten enough to balance their insulin intake. Consequently, the insulin forces the blood sugar level down. The individual first becomes confused, then weak and unable to stand, and can eventually go into a coma.

Most sufferers are warned about the signs and often have a boiled sweet or a lump of sugar handy as a quick means of keeping up their blood sugar level until they can have a proper meal.

First Aid

A diabetic coma needs special treatment in a hospital to bring the blood sugar level down and correct the bodily disturbance with an intravenous drip.

Immediate attention to a hypo-glycaemic crisis is needed, while the patient is still conscious. Give them a small sugary drink. And once they are thinking clearly they will know precisely what to do, having been well instructed. They will often have the pre-prepared glucose injection at home which can be given, after instruction, by a relative or friend.

DIARRHOEA

Most attacks of diarrhoea are caused by gastro-intestinal infections – think of them as the body's way of getting rid of harmful substances. If your diarrhoea is accompanied by vomiting, food poisoning is also a likely cause. A viral infection generally known as gastric flu could be the culprit, too. Fortunately, the diarrhoea is usually over before investigations are necessary.

Another common cause of diarrhoea is stress. It can be a side-effect of taking certain drugs – antibiotics, for example. Tetracycline, and other commonly prescribed 'broad spectrum' antibiotics, can destroy friendly bacteria which normally live in the bowel and are part of our natural defences against more harmful bacteria. Consequently, if they are destroyed, the harmful ones – perhaps resistant to the antibiotic – can thrive. But if this happens to you, don't just stop taking the antibiotics. Ring your doctor and ask for advice.

Signs and Symptoms

Symptoms of diarrhoea are loose or liquid bowel movements, often accompanied by cramping pain in the lower abdomen.

First Aid

Whatever the cause, most attacks of diarrhoea usually clear up quickly and without medical attention. The best way to treat it is not eating for twenty-four hours and drinking plenty of watery drinks. See also Holiday Tummy, page 221.

> **BE CAREFUL!**
>
> The greatest risk from diarrhoea, and from vomiting too, is that the body's essential minerals are lost at the same time, which can lead to dehydration. The very young and the elderly are particularly at risk. (See also Dehydration, page 89.)

DISLOCATIONS

Dislocations are injuries commonly to shoulders, thumbs, fingers and jaws. The usual meaning of a dislocation is a bone that has become wrenched out of place at a joint.

🛈 Signs and Symptoms

Warning signs to look out for are very bad pain, swelling over the injured area as well as bruising. Movement is likely to be very difficult.

➕ First Aid

In fact, the symptoms of a dislocation are similar to those of broken bones, and you must seek medical treatment if you suspect a dislocation. Certainly don't try to perform any do-it-yourself remedies. You'll need to try to keep the injured area immobile, and follow the advice given under Broken Bones, page 51.

DIZZINESS

Dizziness is an extremely common condition. In young people, it's often brought on by anxiety or an emotional problem, although, of course, their GP will examine them thoroughly to make sure that there's no physical cause. When dizziness strikes older people out of the blue, there's more likely to be a physiological reason (for example, abnormal heart rhythms).

As many as one in five women experience a whole range of often distressing symptoms, including dizzy spells, at the menopause. Hormone Replacement Therapy is suitable for many women – it reduces the symptoms and offers protection from the bone-thinning disease, osteoporosis.

For many others, however, the cause remains unidentified, but it is likely to be due to a whole range of mild, but distressing, malfunctions in the body's natural systems.

Keeping our balance requires a complex combination of information from our eyes and nerves, which tells our brain where we feel we are in relation to the ground. The brain transmits messages at the same time to make one group of muscles relax while others contract, keeping us steady.

Over and above this – and in particular when our eyes are shut – the balance mechanism in our inner ear feeds a mass of information into our brain about our position in space.

Given that this highly sophisticated mechanism, which a modern computer would be proud of, can be affected by our moods, our hormones and our emotional life, it's hardly surprising that from time to time it can get out of order, without any precise medical explanation being obvious.

➕ First Aid

Dizziness can be very distressing. Sufferers have described it as similar to being extremely sea-sick in a force 10 gale.

If you suddenly feel dizzy make sure you get yourself out of any position of danger – away from an open fire or dangerous machinery, for example. If you think you are going to faint either lie on the floor or put your head between your knees (see page 114).

Fortunately, most of the people who have severe vertigo find that medicines like Stemetil will dampen down their symptoms.

✒ Prevention

These drugs don't offer a long-term solution to the problem and, in fact, can make matters worse. Many sufferers with symptoms turn to relaxation and alternative therapies just to see if there's some non-medical way to bring relief.

It is worth remembering, too, that most patients suffering from unexplained dizziness find it does get better as the years pass.

DOG BITES

When you're bitten by a dog you need to seek professional medical advice because in all likelihood you'll require an anti-tetanus injection. See Tetanus Jabs, page 22.

Signs and Symptoms

Dog bites usually cause deep puncture wounds and therefore any infection that is introduced cannot readily be washed away by water or by the body's own cleaning mechanism, bleeding. However, a bite from a healthy dog is not likely to be much worse than any other deep wound, so similar advice applies (see page 178).

First Aid

If you are bitten try to rinse the affected area under running water at the sink. Then wash the wound as thoroughly as you can, using soap and water. Dry the area gently using a clean

---

Rabies

In many developing parts of the world, rabies is the great fear following a dog bite. The virus causes the dog to behave in a wild, uncontrolled way, readily biting people and other animals. Rabies in humans is a dread disease eventually causing intense muscle spasms, particularly of the throat when trying to drink (or even when thinking about drinking). If you are bitten by an animal that is thought to be rabid, preventative injections can now be given immediately which can stop the virus developing.
In Europe and other parts of the developed world, where rabies still exists, most dogs are immunised against it. Consequently it is now rare in these countries.

---

cloth. For a minor wound cover with a plaster or a suitable dressing. If the wound is bleeding, let it bleed for up to a minute, unless it is already bleeding heavily, in which case apply pressure and if possible raise the injured limb. You'll then need to get yourself off to your doctor's surgery or hospital.

If you have reason to think that the dog is a stray or running wild, you should report it to the police.

DROWNING

If you inhale water instead of air the consequences are dire. If a person who is in danger of drowning is pulled from the water quickly there is a chance that they can be saved.

⊕ First Aid

If you think that someone is drowning get to them as quickly as you can but bear in mind your own safety and those of others who might need to risk their lives to save you. Too often there can be two or three tragedies instead of the one that would have taken place without intervention. Jumping into a raging sea when you can't swim is not going to help anyone.

However, once you've reached the person in difficulties, try to get them breathing again before you get them out of the water. Use the technique for removing an object from the windpipe (see page 69).

⬤ Prevention

Be aware of the dangers of drowning where children are concerned. A child can drown in only two inches of water.

My wife (a trained nurse) and I have between us resuscitated three people who had been pulled from the water while bathing, either not breathing (two) or not breathing and pulseless (one). I'm proud to say we saved all three, although the last one had to be admitted to hospital overnight before he was given a clean bill of health.

Take great care when a child is near water, be it the sea or a garden pond. Don't ever leave a baby or toddler alone in a bath or bathroom – don't forget that even certain lavatories could pose a threat to a young child whose head could become submerged in the water if you weren't around. And, better still, try to teach them to swim as soon as you can.

DRUGS AND OVERDOSES

Drug abuse can take many forms. The following list covers the commonest drugs sold illegally.

✷ Relaxants

Cannabis: one of the most common of the illegal drugs. It can be smoked. Sold as a solid dark brown resin, it is crumbled, mixed with tobacco and then smoked. The effects it produces are those of relaxation, the user becoming very talkative and in a state of intoxication.

✷ Stimulants
All stimulants affect the nervous system.

Amphetamine: can be sniffed or injected. It is dangerous particularly for those people who have any kind of heart condition as it can overstimulate the heart. In excessive dosage or with a pre-existant illness it can cause heart and circulatory failure.

Cocaine and **Crack:** cocaine is mostly sold in powder form and is usually sniffed but it can also be injected. Crack looks like a raisin-sized crystal. It is smoked. It is a cheap alternative to cocaine. Both are drugs of addiction. The main dangers, except in large 'toxic' dosage, are social ones related to the need to get the drugs (in other words, the criminality that goes with it).

Ecstasy: sold in the form of a tablet or coloured capsule, it's very dangerous for those with heart conditions, high blood pressure, mental problems or those who suffer from epilepsy.

✳ Hallucinogens, tranquillisers and sedatives

LSD: also known as acid, it is sold in tablet form and its effects range from a feeling of elation to wild hallucinations.

Tranquillisers and **sedatives:** sold in tablet form, their effects vary depending on the type and dosage. For many people they relieve anxiety, remove social inhibitions and provide a 'spaced out' feeling. They are drugs of dependance and even addiction. They are considered drugs of abuse when they have not been specifically prescribed for medical conditions.

✳ Heroin

Perhaps surprisingly to many people who have not come into contact with drug users, heroin addicts can control their symptoms (moodiness, irritability and extreme restlessness, for example) as long as they can maintain supplies of the drug. Nevertheless with very high doses chronic sedation can occur.

Heroin is the dried 'milk' of the opium poppy and in its pure form it's a white powder with twice the strength of morphine. Compared with other opiates, heroin is effective, acts quickly, is easy to dissolve in water for injection, and causes fewer side-effects like vomiting. To produce an effect opiates must be absorbed into the bloodstream. Most opiates, including heroin, are only poorly absorbed from the stomach after swallowing. Heroin is much more effective if it's sniffed, smoked or injected, so misusers will generally use these methods rather than 'waste' the drug by swallowing it. When sniffed, heroin is absorbed into the bloodstream via the nose as it soaks into the porous nasal lining.

When smoked the heroin is drawn into the lungs, quickly entering the bloodstream. 'Chasing the dragon' is a way of smoking heroin by heating the powder and inhaling the fumes through a small tube. Heroin can also be injected into the bloodstream through a vein – the effects are almost immediate and stronger as none of the drug is lost before entering the bloodstream.

Prevention of drug addiction
The initial causes of drug addiction can be social depri-
vation as well as having a very unhappy childhood. But it
can also sometimes stem from opportunity – coming
into contact with a ready supply of cannabis, cocaine,
ecstasy or heroin and trying it for kicks. There's no
doubt that heroin is truly addictive. It destroys lives as
well as life itself. Often, the treatments available are
compromises and none are straightforward or ideal.
Sufferers must have self-restraint and they need constant understanding, care and attention in return.
Education to promote an awareness of the great risks of
drug taking is only one means of prevention. The other
is the control of opportunity – and that's a job for everyone, not just the police.

🛑 Signs and Symptoms

The signs and symptoms of drug taking can be numerous
and depend on the type of drug that has been taken. A person
can appear over-stimulated, talkative, behave as if drunk, suffer
sedation, have hallucinations or lose consciousness.

In children, an unexpected change in behaviour – telling
lies out of character, acting strangely, becoming withdrawn and
secretive to a worrying degree – are signs to be aware of.

➕ First Aid

If you think someone has been taking drugs and is unconscious, keep calm and carry out the following procedures.

1 If they have stopped breathing, give mouth-to-mouth
   resuscitation (see page 16). Make sure they've got fresh
   air.
2 Turn them on their side and put them in the recovery
   position (see page 18). This is an essential position
   because it will help prevent them inhaling any vomit as
   the head is slightly lower than the rest of the body.
3 Dial 999 and ask for an ambulance.

4 Collect up any evidence around them that shows what they might have been doing – their 'works', any powders, syringes, etc. – and give them to the ambulance driver.

5 Take care to avoid pricking yourself or others with any needles – called needlestick injuries – as these can carry infection, particularly the Hepatitis B, HIV and other viruses.

For accidental overdose of medicines see Swallowing Poisons, page 204, and for glue sniffing see Solvent Abuse, page 185.

EARACHE

Otitis media is, put simply, a painful infection of the middle ear. It's the type of infection that young children are particularly prone to because their natural antibodies are not yet fully developed. Also, the Eustacian tubes which connect the back of the nose to the middle ear chamber on either side are shorter and more horizontal than they will be in adulthood. Both of these factors allow germs to enter the middle ear more readily in childhood.

Sometimes a child can wake in the night with terrible earache which is relieved by paracetamol. In the morning there may be traces of blood on his or her pillow but the earache has gone. Whatever the cause, a doctor's examination is essential. Such an occurrence could have been something as straightforward as an infected pimple in the outer part of the hole leading down to the ear, which is occasionally subject to small boils.

But earache in a child is most often due to an infection or congestion in the middle ear, just inside the eardrum. In an acute attack, the pressure can build up quickly so that the drum is perforated (see page 174). This automatically releases the tension and the pain usually goes at the same time. If this is the case, your doctor would want to keep an eye on it and would want to prescribe antibiotics to be sure.

What about antibiotics?
Are antibiotics always needed for earache? Sometimes antibiotics are prescribed as a safeguard even though they do not combat viral infections, responsible for a high proportion of such problems. But when it comes to ear infections, it's not always easy to establish whether or not it is viral or bacterial.

❗ Signs and Symptoms

When a child is too young to speak, they may cry, hold their ear and have a raised temperature.

➕ First Aid

When a child wakes in the night with earache, the best thing you can do is reassure him. Give paracetamol suspension in the recommended doses. Gentle heat may also ease the pain, but if you give a child a hot water bottle to hold against the ear, make sure you wrap it in a towel first and that it is not too hot.

Ear infections like otitis media are treated with paracetamol to ease pain and also by the use of decongestants or antihistamines to reduce any swelling in the Eustachian tube. This enables any pus to come out of the middle ear. So in the morning arrange an appointment with your doctor.

EARS, FOREIGN OBJECTS IN

Children can – and do – push things into all sorts of unexpected places!

❗ Signs and Symptoms

The first you may know of such an incident will be a discharge coming from the ear or yells of pain.

Ear wax

While talking about ears, a word of advice. Everyone has a certain amount of wax in their ears – it is a natural substance secreted by tiny glands in the skin of the ear similar to sweat glands. It helps protect the sensitive lining in the outer channel of the ear from infection and keeps it free of dust and flakes of skin. And just as some people sweat more than others, some people naturally produce more ear wax.

Usually the wax crumbles away steadily and is expelled as tiny flakes, to be replaced by a fresh supply of wax from within the ear. It only becomes troublesome when there is a build-up of too much wax, which, if left for a long time, may harden or slip against the drum and cause hearing problems.

I must urge you to take great care with your ears – never delve inside too deeply or you could damage the drum, and never scratch the skin lining the hole as this may cause inflammation.

⊕ First Aid

If your child has something lodged in the ear, or in the rare instance that an insect has made its way into the ear, don't try to remove it yourself, but get medical help as quickly as possible because any ear injuries caused could result in loss of hearing. See your doctor who will be able to look into the ear with an instrument called an auroscope, which will help him establish exactly where the foreign object is lodged. Quite often he or she will be able to syringe the object out. If he can't he is likely to refer the child to an ENT surgeon who has the right instruments to pick it out under direct vision.

WARNING

Do not attempt to clean or unblock your ears with cotton wool buds, nor force instruments into the ear.

ELECTRIC SHOCK

When you think a person has had an electric shock turn off the power source at the mains before you do anything else. Don't touch the person with bare hands (especially wet ones) unless you are absolutely sure that the electric current has been turned off. They will probably still be touching the appliance that gave them the shock so you must move that out of their grasp by using a wooden implement such as a broomstick if you have any doubts about the current being on. Also you'll need to find some newspapers or magazines or a telephone directory to stand on. Then try to separate the casualty from the electric appliance. Paper and wood are not very good conductors of electricity so that should save you from being electrocuted too.

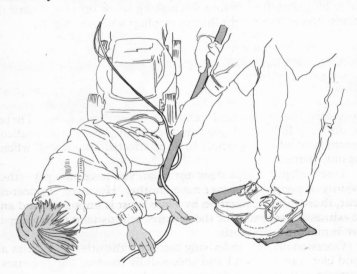

❗ Signs and Symptoms

Warning signs that someone might have had an electric shock can be a person lying unconscious near an electrical appliance. An electric shock can stop the heart beating or it can cause severe burns.

✚ First Aid

Check the pulse. If it is absent, begin heart massage (see page 13). If the person is not breathing give mouth-to-mouth resuscitation (see page 16) immediately. Once they are breathing again, place them in the recovery position. Call for help. If the casualty has suffered from burns deal with these also (see page 59).

🚫 Prevention

Make sure all electrical appliances are wired correctly and replace worn-out fittings and frayed flexes. Disconnect all appliances before doing any repair jobs on them and remove the appropriate fuse before attempting work on any electrical circuit. Never touch light fittings or plugs with wet hands.

EPILEPTIC FITS

Epilepsy is a pattern of fits or seizures caused by an abnormal discharge of electric energy from the brain. Sufferers experience short episodes of changed behaviour or consciousness. There are differing forms and degrees of epilepsy. The fits are called 'generalised' when the whole brain is affected; and 'focal' when it is only partial.

One epileptic attack does not mean you have epilepsy – the majority of people will never have another. However, if seizures recur, thorough investigation by a specialist is important and an eye-witness description of the seizures will usually play a large part in making a diagnosis.

Occasionally, an underlying cause for the attacks, such as a blood clot, can be found and successfully treated. Other causes of attacks include brain damage at birth, meningitis, and severe concussion.

Certain triggers, such as flashing lights or even a heavy bout of drinking, can also bring on a fit in some people. Usually, there is no apparent cause, though there is an inherited tendency to epilepsy – for example, if one parent has the condition their children have a one in forty chance of developing it. If both parents have it, the chance becomes one in four. In most instances, however, there is no past history of epilepsy in the family.

Symptoms vary and range from the almost unnoticeable 'absences' (which used to be called 'petit mal') – common in childhood and often mistaken for daydreaming – to a major 'tonic-clonic' attack (previously called 'grand mal') when convulsions occur. In other types of seizure, people may go into a trance-like state (different to absences), perform repetitive actions such as lip-smacking or experience strange smells and tastes.

Fortunately, most people who suffer from epilepsy are able to control their fits completely with appropriate drugs. These anti-convulsant drugs help neutralise excessive electrical activity in the brain. Specialists are able to use precisely the right amount of medication, now that they can monitor its concentration in the body by blood tests.

❗ Signs and Symptoms

Signs that a person is having an epileptic fit are a sudden loss of consciousness, uncontrolled body movements such as twitching or shaking or frothing at the mouth.

✚ First Aid

To watch someone having a seizure with convulsions, if you know nothing about epilepsy, can be frightening. Under-

---

Let's put the record straight

I would just like to put the record straight while talking about epilepsy. No objects should be jammed into a sufferer's mouth while he or she is having a fit as, during the seizure, the person cannot swallow or spit out anything, which is why saliva spills out. If a bit of tooth is chipped off by inserting an object into the mouth, this can go down into the lungs and be life-threatening. Trying to restrain their jerking movements is likely to result in dislocated joints for the sufferer and harm to yourself.

---

standably, people often panic, and, in their wish to help, do the wrong thing. Don't, for example, push something into their mouth to stop them biting their tongue. It can smash teeth which may be sucked down the windpipe. This is far more serious than a bitten tongue, which is unlikely to occur anyway.

Most helpful, in fact, is to do very little except be calm and reassuring and stay with the person while the fit runs its course. It will probably last about five minutes.

If they are in danger – lying in the road, for instance – move them to a safe place and remove anything on which they could hurt themselves. Turn the sufferer on to his or her side in the recovery position once the convulsions have stopped.

Unless the fit lasts more than five minutes, or is followed by another, it should not be necessary to call medical help.

Once the attack has passed the person may feel a drowsy and confused and will appreciate help to get home. Often, though, they recover quickly and – especially if they are used to having attacks – prefer not to be fussed over. False prejudices about epilepsy and worries about how others will react to an attack can be more upsetting to the sufferer than the fits themselves.

EYE INJURIES

The aim of dealing with any eye emergency is to prevent further damage to these very delicate organs. If you are dealing with someone who has damaged an eye it is essential that they *do not rub it*.

Cuts to the eyes are serious, but modern advances in surgical techniques mean that many injuries can now be repaired successfully.

🛈 Signs and Symptoms

Signs that an eye has been injured include:

* pain
* the eye can look bloodshot
* there may be loss of vision
* the eye could leak some clear fluid, the aqueous humour from the front of the eye

First Aid

If you think someone has injured their eye, immediately seek medical help. If in doubt about the severity, call an ambulance.

If you have to bandage an injured eye, always bandage both eyes, otherwise the injured eye continues to work and move with the good one.

EYELASH IN THE EYE

Eyelashes do sometimes fall into the eye and cause irritation and discomfort.

Signs and Symptoms

Mild pain or discomfort in the eye. When you look in a mirror you'll usually be able to see the offending lash.

First Aid

The best way to remove an eyelash which has dropped into your eye – if you feel it is below your bottom lid – is to look in the mirror and pull down the lower lid gently by pulling the skin from half an inch below it. With the corner of a clean handkerchief carefully wipe the eyelash away.

If the eyelash is below the top lid, you cannot see it but you feel it is there, you can seek the advice of your local pharmacist. He or she will be able to supply you with an eye bath and a sterile eye solution. Some pharmacists will remove a lash from below the top eyelid for you. It's likely that the top lid will have to be everted (flipped outwards) and the lash wiped away with a clean brush kept for that purpose or the corner of a sterile cloth.

EYES, FOREIGN OBJECTS IN

First Aid

If an object is embedded into the eye do not attempt to remove it. If you can, cover the injured eye with an eye pad. (As

I said opposite, cover both eyes, because if the casualty can still see, and is therefore moving one eye, the injured eye will automatically move too, possibly damaging it further.) Seek medical help urgently.

For simpler problems, such as a tiny thread of cotton wool in the eye, pulling the upper lid over the lower lid by holding on to the eyelashes can help, or bathing the eye with cool, previously boiled water, using a clean eggcup if you don't have an eye bath.

For other vision problems, see Focusing Difficulties (page 120) and Glaucoma (page 125).

FAINTING

Fainting is a natural occurrence when not enough blood is getting to the brain. A faint causes a person to fall to the floor and, as it no longer has to 'push' against gravity, the blood immediately floods the brain again. It's nature's way of sorting out the problem, if you like.

Elderly people can faint because of a heart irregularity. In the young and fit fainting can happen as a result of standing in one position for too long. It takes place during pregnancy because very often the blood pressure is lower than normal.

Take your time

Fainting in the morning may be caused by leaving for work in a great rush without having anything for breakfast. If your last meal was quite early the previous evening, that's a long time to go without food and the amount of glucose (sugar) – essential for energy – circulating in your blood would therefore be low. Fainting is nature's way of making you lie down to allow more oxygen and nutrients to reach your brain. Morning faints are very common, particularly in young women and those on diets. Get up a little earlier and make sure you at least have a bowl of cereal and some toast before you leave home.

❗ Signs and Symptoms

Someone about to faint often feels unwell and light-headed first, but sometimes you may simply find yourself waking up on the floor.

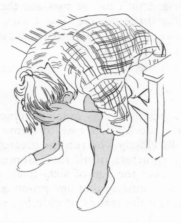

➕ First Aid

You can help a person who has fainted by lifting their feet slightly off the floor to help the blood flow to the brain. If an individual faints while they are in a sitting position, so that the body can't fall to the floor, then they must be helped to the floor or the head bent forward between the knees.

FALLS IN A CHILD

Children often fall while they are running or playing. They can become excited or reckless or lose concentration on what they are doing and its safety aspects.

❗ Signs and Symptoms

When children fall they usually end up with bumps on the head, or cuts and grazes.

✚ First Aid

To help take the pain away you must apply something cold, such as a flannel soaked in cold water that has been well wrung-out. When applied immediately this will help to numb the pain and reduce bruising. Don't rub or massage the bruised area – pressure may make things worse. For a cut, clean the area under running water, or gently wipe with antiseptic or a piece of cotton wool soaked in warm water.

FALLS IN THE ELDERLY

The frequency of accidents is very much governed by a person's age. Children have the highest rate of home accidents, for example, yet it is the elderly who run the greatest risk of a fatal one (almost three-quarters of all fatal home accidents are suffered by people over the age of sixty-five). And the major type of home accident among that age group is a fall of some kind. Each year many thousands of elderly people fall down stairs.

The older you are the more likely you are to fall. Regrettably, you're also more likely to fracture the thigh bone – the femur – and this may be the last straw. It puts the old person in hospital and, since the femur is the largest bone in the body and the operation to pin it is a major procedure, it's just too much for the body to stand.

More serious injuries, which I must point out are less frequent than minor injuries, may involve concussion or a fracture, often of the wrist and hip. In older women it can often be the hip, wrist, upper arm and pelvis. Head injuries can occur if a person falls down stairs, for example, or hits their head on the corner of a radiator.

✳ Osteoporosis: a problem of age

Osteoporosis, a thinning of the bones, can cause painful fractures. With this condition, bones become brittle, cannot withstand the wear and tear of everyday activities and so break easily. Indeed, sufferers who fracture a hip often believe a fall has caused it when, in fact, it's more likely that the weight of

115

> *Be prepared*
> Falls for a person living on their own can prove a problem. Consequently, I'm a great believer in alarms which can be hung around the neck and, when pressed, will ring a prearranged person's telephone, letting them know that help is needed.

the body alone was enough to bring about the fracture, which then caused them to trip and stumble. Similarly vertebrae can crumble without any cause if they are badly weakened by osteoporosis.

Women after the menopause are particularly prone to thinning of the bones. As many as one in four post-menopausal women is likely to develop osteoporosis compared with less than one in forty men of that age. Men have a denser bone structure than women which makes them less at risk, and they don't have the dramatic reduction of the hormone oestrogen that women undergo during the menopause. This hormone is particularly important in cases of osteoporosis because it helps the body to absorb the calcium it needs for the maintenance of strong, healthy bones.

Half of the women over the age of seventy-five will develop osteoporosis. Small, fair, thin-boned women are particularly at risk, and unfortunately it does run in families because mothers and sisters are likely to be of similar build.

➕ First Aid

Most injuries as a result of a minor fall or stumble will include soft tissue injuries, such as bruises or sprains and strains. In this case you will need to apply a cold compress to the injured area. For more information about bruises, see page 57. Other injuries are likely to include cuts and grazes. See pages 27 and 84.

Capsulitis, an inflammation of all the tissues around a joint – its capsule, hence the name – can affect elderly people after they have had a fall, though the onset of symptoms is usually several hours later.

After a fall, you'll need to watch out for signs such as

swelling or pain which may indicate a fracture. For more information on fractures see Broken Bones, page 51.

Sometimes a mild headache can follow if an elderly person has knocked his or her head. But should the pain persist a doctor's advice will need to be sought to rule out any other causes. If a person has fallen and has lost consciousness, even if only for a few seconds, he may suffer from concussion (see page 76). If after a fall a person becomes confused, albeit mildly and immediately following the accident, then it may not be too much cause for alarm, as bruising to the brain can lead to this state of mind. But a more exaggerated form of confusion can be a sign of something much more serious, such as internal bleeding in the skull. Any worrying symptoms after a fall mean the person must be seen by a doctor.

Prevention

Fear of falling can make you lose confidence and some people find that they don't want to go out very often and so become increasingly housebound just because they are frightened of tripping, particularly during the winter months when pavements are very slippery.

One way of preventing falls is to look around your home to assess what could be a risk or a potential danger zone, and try to do something about it sooner rather than later. Secure carpets that are not fitting properly (particularly those on stairs), and rugs or mats (often actually called slip mats!) that could cause someone to trip up. Make sure that all shoes fit you and are properly laced.

FEBRILE CONVULSIONS

Some children may have a convulsion or fit – known as a febrile convulsion – if a raised temperature is severe enough. This can be dangerous, as well as alarming for both the parents and the child. The typical age range during which a child may have a febrile convulsion is six months to three years.

It is perfectly understandable that, whenever a baby or a child has a fit, the parents get worried. But it may help them to know that as many as one child in twenty will have a fit before they reach the age of five, purely as the result of a high temperature.

If there is no history of fits in the family, or if the fit is over quickly – generally within about three minutes – and especially if the child is under one year of age, then the chances of him or her having another one are reduced.

Likewise, while virtually every child is likely to fit if his or her temperature is very high – 104°F/40°C or above – if yours has experienced a febrile convulsion as a result, they are reasonably unlikely to have another. This is because temperatures at that level are very rarely reached in an otherwise healthy child.

So, if a child does fulfil all the conditions mentioned above, then the likelihood of him or her having a second fit is remote. And for those children for whom these details do not apply, the chance of them having another is still only one in three.

The research undertaken that allows such factors to be assessed also arms GPs with the information they need to determine the nature of a fit. They will usually decide to wait to see if the convulsion works itself out spontaneously, confident that the outcome will be a complete recovery. Indeed, by the time a doctor or ambulance arrives on the scene, this has often already happened.

Having said that, of one thing I'm sure: if your baby or child has a fit, don't waste time – having made sure of his immediate safety (see First Aid, below) always consult a doctor.

🛈 Signs and Symptoms

The signs of a fit will be obvious – the child's body, or sometimes just a limb, may become rigid, then relaxed and then rigid again, and so on. The child's face may become contorted and his mouth be tightly shut with teeth clenched.

➕ First Aid

If your child is having a febrile convulsion there is not much you can do except wait for it to end. Let the fit run its course and do not hold them down or stop their limbs from moving as you could cause them more injury this way. However, do stay with them to make sure they do not hurt themselves or choke on vomit. Once the fit is over, put them into the recovery position (see page 18), then report it to your doctor. If it continues for more than a couple of minutes phone him or her for advice.

FEVER

A fever can be a symptom of any one of several illnesses, but is usually a sign that your body is fighting infection. Coughs, colds and other infections are often accompanied by aches, pains and feverishness.

🛈 Signs and Symptoms

A high temperature (over 38°C/100.4°F) which makes you sweat or shiver.

➕ First Aid

To help reduce a fever, take the recommended dose of aspirin, ibuprofen or paracetamol. As the body will be losing water due to perspiration dehydration needs to be prevented, so drink plenty of cold, alcohol-free fluids. Remember feverish babies or children also need plenty to drink. Don't worry unduly if they do not want to eat or they want to sleep more than usual. Sleep is nature's way of resting the body.

✳ Fevers in children

I'm often asked about whether people with fevers, especially children, should be kept warm. I once received a letter about an on-going argument between a young mother and her mother-in-law. The mother thought that if someone has a fever it's best not to cover them in layers of blankets. Her mother-in-law insisted the opposite was true. So which of them was right?

Well, young children are prone to very high temperatures that occur quite suddenly. Modern teaching says that when the temperature is severe and the child feels very hot, it's as well to keep them uncovered in a comfortably cool – but not cold – room of even temperature, and bathe their body with a flannel or sponge moistened with lukewarm water. You can give a baby a bath in tepid water. As the water evaporates from the hot surface of the body, it produces a cooling effect. However, when the temperature comes down as the body cools, the patient will need to be covered up again. When the temperature is as high as 40°C/104°F, phone your doctor for advice.

FOCUSING DIFFICULTIES

People ask me whether it's normal for someone in their fifties to have difficulty focusing early in the day and late at night. This is a very common problem for people in their middle or later years. The reason is that the intra-ocular muscles, which control the eye's lens, lack tone first thing in the morning when you awake, and in the evening they can slacken again as you become gradually more tired. Coupled with this, the eye lens itself generally tends to become stiffer as we get older, causing less accurate vision from time to time.

BE CAREFUL!

You can never be too careful with eyes. Some serious eye disorders can cause a sudden blurring of vision, so if you experience any problems with your vision it is best always to consult your doctor. Acute glaucoma, for example, is a particular problem for those in their middle or later years (see page 125).

FOOD POISONING

See Diarrhoea, page 97.

FROSTBITE

You develop frostbite when you are exposed to severe drops in temperature. The extreme cold can cause the blood to stop flowing to that area of the body and so the skin becomes frozen. The body does this to preserve its heat so that vital, usually central, organs can continue to function. That's why the extremities such as fingers, toes, ears and nose are the areas of the body most at risk.

⊕ Signs and Symptoms

If frostbite is developing a person will experience pins and needles in the extremities and the affected part will lose colour as the area becomes numb. The skin will then begin to look blue and even black.

⊕ First Aid

Frostbite must be treated quickly. Your first action is to warm the affected areas very slowly. Hold the sufferer's hands in your hands if they are warm, or against a warm part of your body, or place the hands or feet in only just warm, not hot (not more than body temperature) water. Painkillers may be needed to relieve any pain. When the conditions have been extreme or the individual's body temperature has started to fall, seek medical help at the same time.

FROZEN SHOULDER

A frozen shoulder is an acute inflammation that can cause a lot of pain, especially with movement.

⊕ Signs and Symptoms

If it affects the whole joint, any movement in that shoulder will be excruciating. So, when a doctor examines it by pressing with the tips of his fingers, he won't necessarily find any one point that's much more tender than the rest.

The whole joint isn't always affected, however. Sufferers who experience pain only when they try to move their arm above the waist have what's known as the painful arc syndrome. This is due to an inflamed point on the top of the shoulder where the tendon of the supra spinatus muscle acts like a pulley to raise the arm. When a doctor examines the shoulder, he'll find an acutely tender spot where the tendon has become inflamed, but if he lifts the now passive arm, it won't hurt – it only hurts when the patient tries to raise it themselves and the inflamed tendon 'grates' in its 'pulley'.

When the sufferer, rather than the doctor, uses the good arm to raise the other one to shoulder level, he or she will normally find that the affected arm can now take over, without help. So the 'arc' of movement from the waist up to shoulder height is hindered because of pain.

✚ First Aid

When the joint as a whole is affected, rest and anti-inflammatory medicines alone may cure the inflammation. Ice packs or gentle heat applied to the area may help to ease pain. By rest, I don't mean total immobility, however. You will still need to keep your shoulder in motion by moving it with care, holding your arm with your 'good' arm to help it through its normal range of movement. You can ask someone else to do this for you if you prefer.

But, if it's still as bad after a week or so, then passive exercises – gentle manipulation by a physiotherapist, for example – may be recommended to ease the pain and get the joint moving properly again. Your doctor will be able to advise you on the best course of treatment to take.

If there's just a tender spot – at the supra spinatus tendon, for example – a single injection of anti-inflammatory medicines into that point can bring speedy relief. In fact, the condition may settle down within forty-eight hours.

Be patient!
Frozen shoulders sometimes persist, causing distressing pain and stiffness, in spite of all the treatments tried. Occasionally, only time seems to bring a cure. A lot of patience is therefore needed, as well as a determination to carry out regularly any recommended exercises to avoid long-term stiffness or weakness of the muscles and bones. There seems to be a 'natural' period of time before the symptoms go completely and this can be anything from three months to two years.

FUME INHALATION

Fumes can be inhaled inadvertently, for example carbon monoxide from a blocked chimney flue, or smoke by a person escaping from a burning building.

🛑 Signs and Symptoms

Apart from unconsciousness, signs of fume inhalation can be coughing and wheezing, headaches, nausea, vomiting, dizziness and stupor.

➕ First Aid

You must get medical help as soon as you can, and in the meantime you must help the casualty breathe freely again. Get them outside in the fresh air so that you don't endanger your own safety. If they do not seem to be breathing you'll need to start resuscitation procedures quickly, see Mouth-to-Mouth Resuscitation (page 16). Then deal with other injuries such as burns or bleeding (see pages 59 and 46). Once an ambulance has arrived the casualty will usually be given oxygen to help overcome any underoxygenation that may be present as a result of the physical effects of the smoke or its gases upon the lungs.

FUNNY TURNS

I remember receiving a letter from a man in his early thirties who had had a 'funny turn' while eating his supper in front of the telly. One minute he was enjoying the programme, the next the food was all over him and the carpet. Such an occurrence could be a faint, a fit, or a 'funny turn'. People who are going to faint will usually feel unwell before they lose consciousness, but that is not always true. Someone may just faint, then on coming round wonder what has happened.

When someone has a fit (as in epilepsy, see page 109) for the first time, he or she too may wonder where they are when they wake up. An irregularity of the heart's rhythm can be enough to cause someone to pass out or feel very strange for a moment or so, though this is more likely to occur in an older person.

It's understandable that people are reluctant to see their GP about this kind of incident. Even if you might be diagnosed as having had an epileptic fit, it's nothing to be ashamed of. What is important is finding out what happened in order to prevent further episodes. You really should discuss any turns or blackouts with your doctor. You might have come to no harm the first time, but such a 'turn' could be disastrous if you were driving or dealing with dangerous machinery.

Sometimes people who go on to have a stroke remember having had what they describe as 'a few funny turns' – for example, weakness in an arm or leg, slurred speech or blurred sight in one eye, lasting a short time and 'not worth bothering the doctor about'. Although these 'little strokes' – which doctors call Transient Ischaemic Attacks (TIA) – are common and only a few sufferers will later have a proper stroke, they should be taken as a warning signal and always be reported to a doctor. Following his examination, appropriate advice or treatment can then be given and a future stroke often prevented.

For first aid advice see Fainting, page 113.

GASHES

See Cuts and Lacerations, page 84.

GASTRIC FLU

See Diarrhoea, page 97.

GASTRO-ENTERITIS

Gastro-enteritis is simply the medical name for food poisoning. Follow the measures outlined under Diarrhoea on page 97.

GERMAN MEASLES

German measles (rubella to give it its official name) is a mild disease but one which causes danger to an unborn baby within the first four months of development. Immunisation against rubella is now offered to all children at around the ages of twelve to eighteen months (usually before fifteen months). See Immunisation Reactions, page 149.

🛈 Signs and Symptoms

Signs of German measles include swelling at the back of the neck and ears, a slight temperature, a runny nose and a rash of fine pink spots. Sometimes symptoms may not even be all that noticeable. The incubation period is about seventeen days.

✚ First Aid

You can treat any child's high temperature with paracetamol which will also help relieve any discomfort.

> **BE CAREFUL!**
>
> If your child or anyone else for that matter has German measles care should be taken to prevent them coming into contact with a pregnant woman, particularly if she is in the first four months of pregnancy. Complications to the unborn baby can include deafness, blindness or even heart or brain damage. A child can pass on the infection a week before the symptoms show, and is infectious for up to five days after the rash has gone.

GLAUCOMA

Glaucoma is caused by a blockage of the normal draining system of the eye which leads to a build up in fluid and therefore pressure. Acute glaucoma is a particular problem for those in their middle or later years.

🛈 Signs and Symptoms

When glaucoma is acute it may cause severe pain in the eye or head, often accompanied by vomiting. At this stage any deterioration of the sight may not have been noticed. Chronic glaucoma can cause a slow loss of sight with few other symptoms. That is why it is so important for those over forty who have had a first-degree relative (father, mother, brother or sister) with glaucoma to have their eyes tested regularly so that it can be stopped in its tracks before any lasting damage is done.

➕ First Aid

Glaucoma can cause blindness, hence the necessity for seeking medical help urgently.

GLUE SNIFFING

See Solvent Abuse, page 185.

GNAT BITES

Reactions to a bite are due to an anti-clotting substance in the insect's saliva which it injects to make the blood – your blood! – flow more easily as it feeds. Although it is not poisonous, this substance can provoke an allergic-type response around the bite and occasionally throughout the body. With gnats (the common name for a mosquito), midges and horseflies it is only the female that bites; she needs the blood in order to rear her young – no consolation to us as we scratch away!

Fortunately, mosquitoes in Britain do not carry disease. When you are bitten early in the season, you are more likely to react and find yourself scratching than later on in the summer. This is because your body gradually develops some tolerance, particularly to your local gnats and midges. However this will not help you when you visit a different area and get bitten by an unfamiliar species!

❗ Signs and Symptoms

Hot, red, swollen, itchy areas of skin.

➕ First Aid

If you have been bitten by a gnat or midge, iced water or witch hazel, calamine lotion or soothing antiseptic creams will usually calm the irritation.

🚫 Prevention

Some people seem to be more attractive to biting insects than others and individuals differ in how much they react. Often you won't feel a bite, but if you've been near inland water on a warm evening wearing short sleeves, a short skirt or shorts, you may well discover swollen areas with tight, shiny skin and a small oozing hole or water blister the next day. Such biting insects don't leave a sting, but can sometimes cause a reaction in sensitive people.

For these people, it's best to avoid any biting insects by staying away from inland water. Bright colours may also attract insects, so wear pale clothes that cover your arms and legs, especially if you seem prone to bites.

In general, insect repellants should protect you for about two hours and if you are bitten and have a bad reaction you can take antihistamine tablets. Try your best not to scratch either bites or stings or you may introduce infection. For a more angry-looking bump your doctor may prescribe antibiotics.

GRAZES

See Cuts and Lacerations, page 84.

GRIT IN WOUNDS

Wounds such as cuts and grazes can easily contain pieces of grit.

➕ First Aid

Whenever you can, wash away any visible grit under a running cold mains tap water. This is one of the most readily

available, clean (virtually sterile) liquids in the house. Its coldness will also encourage the blood vessels to contract and help
to quench the bleeding.

GUNSHOT WOUNDS

Depending on the velocity and construction of the missile, a
gunshot wound may vary between a small puncture hole both
into, through and out of the body, to a highly tissue-destructive
and gaping wound along its pathway.

⊕ First Aid

You'll have to seek medical advice, of course, because a
doctor must ascertain whether any bullet fragments have been
left behind and if they will need surgical removal. In the meantime you can help stem the flow of blood by raising the injured
area if possible and applying pressure to the wound (see Cuts
and Lacerations, page 84). Remember also to treat for shock
(see page 180).

HAMMERED FINGERS

DIY causes countless accidents, not least of which are fingers
being accidentally hit with hammers or mallets.

❗ Signs and Symptoms

Pain, tenderness, bruising of the finger and fingernail.

⊕ First Aid

If you have such an accident you'll need to run your finger
under cold water. The water will help clean any cuts and the
coldness will also numb the pain and help to ease bruising.

If the injury includes a finger or toenail, then the blood can
pool under it without release. As the pressure builds up it will
begin to throb and can be acutely painful. This is called a Sub
Ungual Haematoma and will usually need a doctor's attention

to release the pressure. This is quickly and cleanly achieved when he heats the end of a paper clip until it's red hot. Then, holding the clip in a pair of forceps, he allows the hot end to burn through the nail, releasing the blood and bringing instant relief. If the pain subsides without the need to release the blood, the remaining clotted blood can take many weeks before it is cleared away by the body's cleansing systems.

HANGOVERS

Most of us drink alcohol from time to time without abusing our bodies and damaging our health. Nevertheless, we shouldn't forget that alcohol is a drug which affects the brain and consequently influences our emotions and our behaviour.

Most people like a drink but nobody likes a drunk, so learn your limits and try to stick to them. The same amount of alcohol will affect individuals in different ways – some boisterous, some belligerent, some sleepy. Some seem able to hold their drink better than others, probably because their body's metabolism burns it up quicker (the liver being the organ responsible for this).

❗ Signs and Symptoms

These are well-known and hardly need repeating – hot bloodshot eyes, furry tongue, blurred vision and slow reactions, headaches and a general feeling of being unwell.

➕ First Aid

Nothing cures a hangover – the brain needs time to recover as alcohol is cleared from the system. On average, one unit of alcohol is cleared from the body each hour. So time will be far more effective than any number of cups of black coffee, whose only effect will be to keep you awake and dehydrate you further! But you can make yourself feel better by drinking plenty of water to combat dehydration, taking your preferred painkillers and sleeping it off.

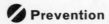 **Prevention**

In future if you have a special night out you can try to limit the effects of a hangover by the following measures. Food slows down alcohol absorption and even a glass of milk or a piece of cheese taken before going out for a drink will help prevent ill effects by 'lining the stomach'. Making your drinks last by sipping them slowly and interspersing each alcoholic drink with a soft drink is a sensible precaution. And I must repeat the wise advice – don't drink and drive.

Drink a pint of water slowly – taking about ten minutes to do so – before going to bed. Next morning drink weak, sweet tea, and as soon as possible go for a brisk twenty-minute walk. Throughout the day avoid natural diuretics such as strong coffee or further alcohol. Stick to bland, non-spicy foods, fresh fruit and vegetables, carbohydrates generally such as pasta, but avoid meat and dairy products. Carbohydrates seem to be gentler on the stomach as they are received more easily than other foodstuffs.

❂ Alcohol abuse

The long-term effects of heavy drinking can cause many medical problems. Alcoholism can cut your life expectancy by ten to fifteen years or lead to drug overdosing, suicide, or accidents and deaths from drunken driving. Too much alcohol can cause:

* blackouts
* serious memory loss
* cirrhosis
* liver cancer
* frequent colds
* reduced resistance to infection
* increased risk of pneumonia and tuberculosis
* puffy eyes
* 'drinker's' nose

Men risk impaired sexual performance or impotence. In women it can lead to unwanted pregnancies and the risk of giving birth to deformed, retarded or low birth weight babies. Not only that, women become dependent on alcohol more quickly than men, seem more liable to liver damage, less responsive to treatment and more prone to ageing, so it is especially important for a woman not to let her drinking get out of hand.

Regular drinking increases a person's tolerance to alcohol. It is possible for someone to consume large amounts daily over a number of years, showing no obvious ill effects or signs of drunkenness, but eventually their health will suffer and they will find they have become dependent on alcohol – unable to do without it. Virtually any symptoms of ill-health may be due to long-term excessive drinking but the most common include:

* frequent stomach pains
* loss of appetite
* irregular or rapid heart beats
* night sweats
* disturbed sleep
* anxiety and/or depression
* forgetfulness
* tingling of fingers or toes

✸ Safe drinking

Alcohol can be enjoyed within reasonable limits. For men the sensible limit is no more than twenty-one units a week and for women it's no more than fifteen (one unit of alcohol equals a half pint of beer or a small glass of wine or a glass of sherry or a single whisky). These are the current nationally supported guidelines though research continues to refine them and we can expect to hear other suggestions as to what, on average, a safe level should be.

Don't forget either that extra strong lagers or beers mean just that. They are probably twice as strong as ordinary types. A pint of ordinary bitter will have the same effect on the body as a double Scotch, as both contain two units of alcohol, although the whisky's effect may be quicker because, up to a certain concentration, the more concentrated the drink, the more rapidly is it absorbed through the stomach lining into the bloodstream. Measures of alcohol served at home are also probably 'stronger' because we tend to pour it in larger amounts than the barman in your local pub.

HEAD INJURIES

Any wound or bump to the head can result in a head injury. Pedestrians, cyclists, drivers, sportsmen, anyone can be at risk of a severe head injury in a serious accident. Skulls can be fractured by a blow to the head, or by a fall. All types of fractures of the skull are dangerous. Apart from any direct injury to or bruising of the brain, damage to its covering membranes can allow the Cerebro Spinal Fluid (CSF) to leak. The seepage of this liquid, which surrounds and cushions the brain, makes it more vulnerable to further damage and the hole through which it is seeping breaches its defences, allowing germs to penetrate inside and take root. Once inside they can readily propagate in this warm, nutrient-rich 'culture', causing massive infection unless treated energetically with antibiotics.

Head injuries can cause brain damage, varying degrees of paralysis, memory loss, difficulties with speech or vision and a complete change of personality. They are a very serious form of injury, which can also endanger life, and need prompt and specialist medical attention.

❗ Signs and Symptoms

Head injuries include concussion (see page 76), a fractured skull and cerebral compression (a serious injury in which bleeding can press on the brain, or cause swelling of the brain, and require surgery).

A fractured skull may be indicated by a part of the skull seeming soft or indented, a loss of consciousness and the casualty being unable to respond well. There may be blood in the whites of the eyes, and blood or clear CSF coming from the apparently undamaged nose or from the ears.

➕ First Aid

Call for medical help and while you are waiting for it to arrive make sure that the casualty is in the recovery position if unconscious, or sitting with head and shoulders raised if alert. If there's bleeding from the scalp, gently exert pressure on the wound with a clean cloth.

HEADACHES

Headaches are an extremely common complaint, afflicting one person in three at least once a year, though some people do tend to suffer more than others. Two of the commonest types of headache are migraine – a severe, recurring headache (see page 161) – and a tension headache, sometimes known as muscle contraction headache.

The tension headache is the most common symptom presented to a general practitioner and no one knows the cause, or why some people get one when they are emotionally upset and some don't.

Other sorts of headache can be triggered by different factors – drinking too much alcohol, sinusitis, anxiety or being in an overheated room or smoky atmosphere. They may be the result of muscle strain in your neck, especially if the headache comes on after you have been reading or doing close work like sewing. You can become tense from concentrating for too long or from sitting in an awkward position.

⚠ Signs and Symptoms

With migraine, the pain is usually one sided and can be accompanied by other symptoms such as loss of appetite, nausea or vomiting. In a tension headache, the whole head throbs and feels as though there's a weight on top of it or a tight band around it. The pain is usually dull and persistent, originating in the muscles of the scalp.

✚ First Aid

First aid for headaches involves taking your preferred painkiller, paracetamol in the case of children, as soon as you feel the headache coming on. Drink plenty of water or other non-alcoholic, clear drinks. Rest in a quiet, darkened room may also be soothing and a warm bath will sometimes relieve tension.

See also Migraine, page 161.

HEAD LICE

Head lice are tiny brown insects with six short, stubbly legs. They're about the size of a pin-head and live on human scalps, laying six to eight eggs a day of a creamy-brown colour. They turn white when the baby louse, called a nymph, has hatched. The remaining pearly white husk is commonly known as a nit, and at this stage is a harmless shell.

The eggs are attached near the base of the hair shaft – a favourite spot is around the ears. Each louse takes two weeks to mature and lives for twenty to thirty days if undetected. The lice feed on blood, using their specially developed mouth-parts to pierce the scalp. They even inject a local anaesthetic into the scalp to prevent their host feeling any pain, and an anticoagulant to stop the blood clotting, thus making it easier for them to feed! They can eventually make your head feel very itchy and worse – hence the well-known phrase 'I feel lousy'! This is because, after about 10,000 bites, your immune system becomes understandably irritated.

Head lice can be a problem among schoolchildren because with them the head louse has never had it so good. We and our children are healthier and cleaner than we have ever been, and the head louse loves it. Clean, healthy heads provide it with the perfect environment.

❗ Signs and Symptoms

Severe itching of the scalp!

To check whether someone has head lice, dampen the hair and then bend the head over a plain sheet of paper. Comb thoroughly to see whether any insects drop out. Then quickly part the hair to look out for moving lice. A magnifying glass will help. You can also see the nits attached to the hair shaft.

✚ First Aid

Your doctor will prescribe one of a variety of lotions or shampoos, but you can also buy some without prescription from your pharmacist.

There are three main insecticides in use that destroy head lice and their eggs – carbaryl, pyrethroids (phenothrin, perme-

> *Did you know?*
> Head lice can't jump or fly, nor do they live in bedding,
> furniture or clothes. The only way they can be passed on
> is by close head contact – a single louse can visit several
> heads in one day just by walking from one to another as
> heads touch during play or an embrace.

thrin) and malathion. They are all equally effective if used as
directed. But health authorities often change their recommenda-
tions for louse treatment preparations every two to three years to
prevent the lice building up a resistance to them.

When applying the shampoo, make sure that no part of the
scalp is left uncovered; pay particular attention to the nape of
the neck and behind the ears.

If a member of your family has head lice, remember to treat
everyone – siblings, parents, grandparents, even lodgers – and
then check them once a week to ensure they're still clear.

Prevention

It is pretty well impossible to prevent children catching lice
from each other. But after treatment you can try to prevent
reinfection. Encourage all your family to comb their hair thoroughly every day, since the female louse – and there are many
more of them than the male – must cling on to two hairs to survive; as combing or brushing separates the hair, the louse will
die and fall off harmlessly. It also breaks the lice's legs, making
them drop off the hair.

HEART ATTACKS

A heart attack or coronary thrombosis occurs when a coronary
artery becomes so severely narrowed that the flow of blood
through it slows down to such an extent that a clot (thrombus)
forms, cutting off the blood supply and completely 'starving'
the section of heart muscle served by that artery. According to
the British Heart Foundation, the heart research charity, it's
estimated that in the UK 300,000 people a year have a heart

attack and it's the commonest cause of early death in the UK (nearly one-third of all deaths of men of working age). Men aged thirty-five to seventy-four in England and Wales are twice as likely to die from coronary heart disease as men in Italy, almost three times more likely than those in France and eight times more likely than those in Japan.

And your chances seem to differ according to where you live within the UK. People in Scotland and Northern Ireland are about 40 per cent more likely to die of coronary heart disease than someone living in the south-east of England. The differences observed between countries and regions are due to variations in both 'race' and lifestyle.

❶ Signs and Symptoms

Generally, someone having a heart attack will have a 'crushing' chest pain, or a pain down their left arm (or both arms), or pain radiating up to their jaw. All three of these symptoms can be present. Although such pains are characteristic of a coronary thrombosis – an acute heart attack – the symptoms are not always so obvious or dramatic.

The person will look greyish and will feel cold and clammy. There will in all likelihood be beads of sweat on their brow.

While the pain of angina may be eased with rest, the pain of a heart attack does not subside on resting. It is said to be one of the most severe pains there is – so much reassurance is needed while waiting for an ambulance.

❶ First Aid

If the person is conscious, he or she should be moved as little as possible and supported in a half-sitting, half-lying position with the knees bent and all tight clothing loosened, while awaiting medical help. If they're awake, give them an aspirin to suck slowly, as aspirin is known to be a powerful clotting prevention agent.

If the patient loses consciousness resuscitation procedures should be followed, see Heart Massage, page 13. Their respiration will also need to be started, see Mouth-to-Mouth Resuscitation, page 16.

✳ Heart disease – some facts and figures

The heart is composed of muscle and, like all muscles, it needs a supply of blood to provide it with nourishment and oxygen. Two main arteries go to the heart and these divide many times to form a network of smaller blood vessels – called the coronary arteries because they resemble a crown – which serve every area of the heart.

Over the years these arteries – and others in the body – can become progressively 'furred up' and narrowed by fatty deposits – or plaques – called atheroma, which build up within them.

Because of these changes in the arteries, the blood flow to the heart can be severely restricted leading to the most common of all the different heart conditions – coronary heart disease (CHD), also known as ischaemic heart disease (IHD).

CHD is a term used to describe narrowing of the blood vessels supplying the heart, the coronary arteries. The most severe form of CHD occurs when a coronary artery becomes blocked – in other words, a heart attack.

◑ Prevention

Although it may not always indicate that a heart problem is developing a common symptom is angina – a tight, gripping pain felt behind the breastbone, sometimes radiating up into the neck or down the left arm. As the arteries become narrower, enough blood may still get through to feed the heart muscle during normal activity but any extra exertion, such as running for a bus, will produce this typical pain which is usually relieved by rest.

If an artery has become extremely narrow, the flow of blood may be slowed to such an extent that it clots. The section of the heart muscle that it serves is therefore cut off from its blood supply and starved of oxygen. The pain will then be like a severe attack of angina but it will not be relieved by rest. This is known as a coronary thrombosis or 'heart attack' and recovery will depend on how large an area of the heart has been affected.

✳ Smoking

Smoking increases your risk of having a heart attack. It's not too late to stop. People who give up smoking are much less likely to have a heart attack than those who continue to smoke.

* A word about fats

Eating too much fat is a risk factor and the chances of you developing heart disease are increased when you are over-weight. This is because sugar, refined carbohydrates and excess animal fat can increase the fats in the blood.

There are three fats in the blood: cholesterol, which comes in two forms – the 'good' type, High Density Lipoprotein (HDL), and the 'bad' type, Low Density Lipoprotein (LDL). The HDL is a kind of transporter fat. It gathers up the LDL and enables it to be safely used by the body. If the ratio of LDL to HDL rises, the excess of LDL gets deposited on the inside of the body's artery walls making them more likely to burst or cause the blood flowing through them to clot. This can cause serious conditions such as a stroke or coronary thrombosis.

Triglycerides are the third fat circulating in the body. High levels of this fat in the blood, while also adding to the problem caused by the LDLs, are specifically associated with inflammation of the pancreas – pancreatitis. This causes a particularly distressing abdominal pain and general malaise. It is very difficult to treat successfully in its chronic form.

Cholesterol is made in the liver; we also take in cholesterol as it is present in most of the animal fats and dairy produce that we eat. Some cholesterol is essential for the normal functioning of the body. But a raised cholesterol level in the blood is one of the most widely recognised causes of coronary artery and other heart conditions. The cholesterol is deposited just under the lining of the heart, its arteries and all the arteries in the body. This restricts the flow of blood and so can cause a heart attack. What's more, it's not only the heart that can be affected. Cholesterol can also weaken the arteries themselves to the extent that they burst. If this happens in the brain, it's called a stroke; if it happens in the big arteries of the heart, it's a dissecting aneurysm.

* Diet

Reducing the level of cholesterol to a normal blood level – especially if it's done in a way that increases the proportion of good cholesterol (HDL) – can reverse much, or all, of the damage that's been done. You can do this by slimming down to your ideal weight, reducing the amount of all fats in your diet, especially the saturated variety (usually of animal origin), and by taking more regular exercise. It's also a good idea to eat proportionately more unsaturated fats and oils – such as olive and corn oils – and also fatty fish – mackerel, herring, and so on – for the unsaturated oil that they naturally contain.

The health benefits of eating fruit and vegetables have been known for quite some time but new research backs results of other studies that state a diet high in beta-carotene and Vitamin E can protect against heart disease and cancer. (Beta-carotene exists in fruit and vegetables – especially carrots. Vitamin E is present in many items of the diet, especially nuts, oils, dairy products, fish and meat.) A report in the *Lancet* told of how researchers from eight countries, including Scotland and Israel, studied 683 men who had suffered heart attacks, compared with 727 healthy controls, to discover whether anti-oxidant vitamins such as beta-carotene and Vitamin E can protect against heart disease. Their results showed that high levels of beta-carotene in body tissue appeared to be protective, but this was not true for Vitamin E. The study also found that the men with the lowest beta-carotene levels were two and a half times more at risk of a heart attack than those with the highest. Men who smoked and who had low beta-carotene levels were most at risk.

✳ High Blood Pressure

High blood pressure means that your chances of coronary heart disease are increased. High blood pressure is a very com-

A few people, about one in 500, are born with a very high cholesterol level due to a particular gene inherited from their mother or father – a condition called Familial Hypercholesterolaemia or FH. The sooner this is diagnosed the better as carefully supervised treatment and a suitable diet can then be given, preferably from childhood onwards, to keep the blood cholesterol at a reasonable level and, hopefully, prevent atheroma and associated problems developing. Unfortunately many do not realise they have FH and the first sign may be a heart attack.

mon problem – something like one in five people are now on
medication for it. A low blood pressure found during a routine
check is usually a health benefit as it indicates the heart and
blood vessels are not under stress, and so the person should live
longer than average as a result.

When your heart beats it causes a surge of blood which
raises the blood pressure. I'm often asked what an abnormal
blood pressure reading is. The first part of the reading denotes
the pressure in the main arteries and heart as they pulse or beat
(systolic). The second reading is the pressure between the beats
(diastolic). Between the ages of fifteen and forty, measurements
ranging from 90/60 to 150/90 can be considered normal when
the person is at rest. A rough easy-to-remember rule is that
normal systolic pressure should generally be no more than 100
plus your age, and the diastolic pressure less than 90.

Blood pressure can increase quite naturally as we get older.
In a middle-aged person, for example, a reading of up to
160/100 could be considered normal enough not to require any
treatment if that person is otherwise fit and healthy.

* Exercise

Lack of exercise too plays a part in heart disease. A recent
national survey by the Sports Council and the Health
Education Authority has revealed that three-quarters of all
adults don't take enough exercise. Yet exercise keeps you in

Did you know?
You may be interested to know that one recent study
found that you need look no further than your fingertips
to tell whether or not you have high blood pressure! A
Medical Research Council study found that the more
whorls people have on the tips of their thumbs or
fingers, the higher their blood pressure and so by impli-
cation the shorter their life expectancy. The explanation
relates back to the formation of the foetus in the womb.
Uncomplicated fingerprints – the arches or loops follow
simple patterns – show that the quality and quantity of
the mother's blood through the placenta was sound.

trim, increases your stamina, helps maintain a healthy heart and is a good means of relieving stress.

But what about those young men who die while exercising? I hear you ask. As it is quite rare for an apparently fit young person who takes plenty of exercise to suffer a heart attack, it does tend to make the news. But out of 1000 fit men who exercise regularly, there will be fewer heart attacks than in 1000 men who don't exercise regularly. That doesn't mean that the first group is risk free, but their chances of having a heart attack are lower.

Whether they exercise or not, it's more likely that those who have an 'early' heart attack will be overweight, smoke, or have had a close relative who also suffered an early heart attack. And it's important that any vigorous exercise is regular. If, for example, a man in his thirties who's heavily overweight and smokes suddenly plays an energetic game of football, then his heart may not be up to it and the sudden strain might cause a heart attack.

✤ Heart failure or heart attack?

What's the difference between heart attacks and heart failure? is another typical question. When one of the arteries to the heart itself suddenly blocks, it's called a heart attack. But when the heart starts to work less efficiently, following a heart attack or for some other medical reason, it's known as heart failure. Heart failure, as the name implies, means that the heart is not working as well as it could, so the blood is not being pumped around the body efficiently. As a result the sufferer may have a build-up of liquid in the tissues, causing swelling of the ankles or, if the person is bed-ridden, in the lower back. The lungs, too, may also collect liquid, since these sites are no longer being drained as efficiently by the bloodstream.

Regrettably, as many as one in 100 people in Britain will be affected by heart failure and it's especially common among the elderly. Fortunately, one of the medicines routinely used to treat blood pressure problems – called ACE inhibitors – will significantly reduce the risk of heart failure following a heart attack, strengthening the heart and reversing many chemical upsets in the body which heart failure can cause.

Who's more likely?
Do men have more heart attacks than women? I am
asked. It's rare for a woman to have angina or a heart
attack before the menopause, which usually occurs
around the age of fifty. Although heart disease is generally seen to be a male problem, after the age of fifty
women do start to suffer from heart problems almost as
often as men.

HEAT ILLNESSES

Heat exhaustion, heat stroke and sun stroke are really quite
similar conditions. They are due to the body overheating,
becoming dehydrated, or the skin becoming burnt. When the
body's heat-controlling mechanisms – the surface blood vessels
opening up to radiate and conduct heat away from the body
and the evaporation of sweat to cool it – are overworked the
enzyme systems may not be able to function so the body's
chemical workings, its metabolism, gives out.

Strenuous exercise in high temperatures can lead to heat
exhaustion as excessive sweating causes a deficiency of salt or
water, or both. With this disruption in the body's fluid balance,
dehydration becomes a real danger.

You don't have to do strenuous exercise to endanger your
body when it comes to heat exhaustion. Excessive sunbathing
can also lead to it. Your internal heat-control mechanism will
try to cool you down by producing sweat which, when it evaporates from the skin, has a powerful cooling effect. When
exposure to the sun is too long, your body can lose too much
fluid in its battle to keep your temperature down, and consequently you can become dehydrated.

🛈 Signs and Symptoms

Warnings of heat exhaustion include headache, dizziness,
nausea, cramps, irritability, confusion, sweating – or a dry skin, a
weak quick pulse or feeling weak. Heat stroke can have additional symptoms of bad sunburn and vomiting, a high temperature
and the person's responses may suddenly become very slow.

✚ First Aid

Heat stroke is more severe and can be fatal if not treated immediately. Get the individual into the cool as soon as possible – into a tepid bath, if one is available, while keeping an eye on him to make sure he doesn't lose consciousness.

Give the sufferer plenty of water to drink to which, ideally, 10 g (¼ oz) of table or cooking salt has been added per 1 litre (1¾ pint).

If someone suffering from a heat illness loses consciousness, follow resuscitation procedures such as mouth-to-mouth resuscitation (see page 16), and then put them in the recovery position (see page 18).

◐ Prevention

Be warned. Heat illnesses can occur in conditions where the sun is weak or even hidden behind clouds. Falling asleep or lying too long in the sun, is, unfortunately, all too common. And the key to avoiding heat illnesses is gradual exposure so your body gets used to the new levels of temperature. This is known as heat adaptation. Wearing a wide-brimmed, white or light coloured hat is also a great help.

See also Sunburn, page 202.

HERNIAS

A hernia occurs when tissue or an organ bulges out of its usual position. The most common sort arises in the groin when some of the abdominal contents squeeze through a hole and protrude into the groin. This sort of hernia, also called a rupture, is more usually found in men, partly because it's often linked to lifting and other strenuous activity but also because men have an extra point of potential weakness where the vessels going to their testicles leave the abdomen.

While men tend to suffer more from a hernia, a hiatus hernia is a lot more common in women (see over page).

🛇 Signs and Symptoms – Hernia

A lump will be felt or noticed in the groin – particularly when coughing or sneezing. There may also be a dragging feeling.

➕ First Aid

If you notice any swelling in the groin, don't try to push it back in yourself. See your doctor to discuss treatment. When a hernia has become strangulated, the swelling can be painful and you may suffer from vomiting. This type needs more urgent medical attention.

🛇 Signs and Symptoms – Hiatus Hernia

The symptoms – a burning sensation behind the breast-bone – arise because part of the stomach is able to 'herniate' upwards into the chest, with the result that the irritant gastric juices can seep through to the gullet. The lining of the gullet, or oesophagus, is not protected against the acids and enzymes of the digestive juices, with the result that it becomes inflamed.

➕ First Aid

If this is happening to you, have a chat with your doctor, as once this condition is diagnosed there are several medicines that can be prescribed to help.

One easy, do-it-yourself aid is to prop up the head of your bed by about six inches. That way the burning juices are less likely to flow upwards.

If you're overweight, a calorie-controlled diet can help, as any excess tissue can press on the stomach and push the acid upwards. For the same reason, when you need to pick up something from the floor, bend from the knees rather than the waist.

HICCUPS

A hiccup is the name given to the characteristic sound caused by an involuntary spasm of the diaphragm which makes the sufferer's chest jump.

Are hiccups ever a cause for worry? They are if they persist. This usually occurs in someone who is very ill or old. Then, the effort needed and the drain on the body's energy reserves can be considerable. For most of us, however, they have come and gone in a very short time.

🛈 Signs and Symptoms

Involuntary gasps of air every few seconds.

➕ First Aid

There are plenty of home remedies for hiccups – drinking from the wrong side of a glass of water, giving someone a fright, holding your breath – though none of these have been definitely shown to work. I believe the best one is just to relax until they go – which is probably what the remedies mentioned above are allowing you to do in any case.

HOUSEMAID'S KNEE

Any continual pressure on a knee joint and kneecap can cause housemaid's knee – known as a prepatellar bursitis.

🛈 Signs and Symptoms

A spongy swelling over or just below the knee.

➕ First Aid

Rest is the best first aid treatment of all. But if any pain or discomfort persists, do see your doctor.

HYPOTHERMIA

When the body's temperature drops below the normal 35–37°C (95–98.6°F), some individuals can suffer from hypothermia, an abnormally low inner body temperature.

hypothermia

❗ Signs and Symptoms

Hypothermia warning signs can be drowsiness, difficulty in speaking, feeling a little wobbly as you try to walk, a puffiness in the face, looking very pale, feeling confused, in addition to the obvious symptom of the skin being very cold to the touch or feeling shivery. It can be a gradual deterioration which means that sometimes a person may not even realise that he or she is at risk.

➕ First Aid

Any casualty on an outdoor expedition needs to be sheltered and kept as warm as possible until help arrives. Cover him or her with a sleeping bag, or blankets, or an anorak, provided this doesn't mean you are putting yourself at risk of over-exposure to cold. A conscious casualty must be offered warm drinks if you have any. If a casualty outdoors, or at home, is unconscious follow resuscitation procedures such as mouth-to-mouth (page 16) while you wait for emergency help.

If you suspect a very young or an elderly person is suffer-

Did you know?

According to a study conducted at the Age Concern Institute of Gerontology, King's College London, elderly people are in 'double jeopardy' during the winter months because they need extra levels of heating in their homes (they spend more time there and their bodies don't work as efficiently as they used to at retaining heat) but are usually less able than younger people to afford it. Consequently, winter is a time of great hardship for many of them, particularly those who live in privately rented accommodation who are less likely to have central heating and good insulation, leading to problems such as dampness, condensation and mould. The survey suggested that three-quarters of a million elderly people could be at risk of developing hypothermia during the winter months and almost a quarter have given up basic necessities like food and clothing to stay warm.

146

ing from hypothermia you must react quickly while trying to warm them in gradual stages. Warm the room, cover them with blankets, give them something to wear on their heads and offer warm drinks. Because the blood circulation just under the cold skin is so sluggish, to apply heat directly in any form is not wise, especially with the very old or very young. The local defences will not be so quick to react and a burn can readily result, even with what would normally be considered only a warm 'hot' water bottle or bath. For sufferers outside those age limits you can suggest they have a warm bath then quickly dress them in warm, dry clothes to prevent any further heat loss from the body. It is advisable to consult a doctor about all cases of hypothermia no matter how old the sufferer.

⏺ Prevention

Each year Age Concern's Coldwatch campaign gives advice on keeping warm.

1 Wrap up warmly before going out, even when it is just to nip out to the newsagent.
2 Remember that several thin layers of clothing are better than one thick layer.
3 Keep warm in bed at night by wearing bed socks and even a hat.
4 If you can't afford to spend much on heating bills, at least try to keep one room warm during cold weather.
5 Consume some hot food and drink each day.
6 Kitchen foil, with the shiny side facing out, fixed on the wall behind central heating radiators, will reflect heat and help to prevent heat being lost.

BE CAREFUL!

Hypothermia can be a problem if you enjoy outdoor expeditions such as hill walking and mountain climbing. Carefully plan each outing, including checking weather reports. Respect the elements in both summer and winter. Wear the correct clothing and always carry a bag containing spare, dry clothes and emergency food rations.

HYSTERIA

True hysteria is the body's unconscious mind taking over its mechanical functions. For example, being unable to move a limb, though when under hypnosis, or anaesthesia and with electrical stimulation, the limb and nerves can be demonstrated to work quite normally.

❶ Signs and Symptoms

Hysteria is a term most people use to describe an individual who finds a social or emotional situation totally unacceptable and screams, cries, hyperventilates or over-breathes (when the breathing rate is obviously high and they are complaining of feeling numb or experiencing pins and needles or cramp in the hand) to the point where they may faint.

Medically, hysteria is also diagnosed when the sufferer has an accentuated physical reaction, such as the inability to move a limb, muscles that 'jump' spasmodically resembling a seizure and many more. As I've said, these phenomena can be shown to return to normal when the patient is hypnotised, for example.

➕ First Aid

Despite all those films in which a hysterical character is slapped across the face, that isn't the course of action you should take when dealing with someone who is hysterical!

Talk calmly to the individual, offer comfort when this is socially acceptable – a proffered hand or holding the arm – or if a family member or friend with a big hug.

Talk calmly to a person who is over-breathing and tell them to blow into a paper bag (it must be paper not plastic or cellophane). The bag must be blown open by them as if to bang it, with the entrance to the bag held loosely over the mouth and nose. This allows the sufferer to re-breathe their expired air which is rich in carbon dioxide, thereby increasing the carbon dioxide content of their bloodstream, which was lowered while the sufferer breathed too quickly.

If you don't have a paper bag, the sufferer can cup his or her hands over the mouth and nose to reproduce the effect.

If the hysteria has resulted in paralysis of a limb, for example, this will obviously require deeper psychological treatment.

IMMUNISATION REACTIONS

Immunisation reactions should not put you off having your child immunised, since thanks to the current immunisation programme it is rare for a child to get diphtheria, tetanus or polio. Incidents of measles, mumps and whooping cough are also becoming fewer as more and more children are immunised. The immunisation programme is the biggest boost there has ever been in the fight against childhood illness and death.

Childhood diseases can be unpleasant and sometimes lethal. As I said, diphtheria and tetanus are now rare in this country only because enough parents have their children vaccinated to keep the viruses in check. Diphtheria begins with a sore throat that can block the nose or throat making it difficult to breathe. Tetanus is caused by germs from soil, dirt or dust getting into an open wound. Fortunately, there's now very little tetanus-related illness except in country areas among certain occupations, such as farm workers, for example, who are at greater risk. Polio, which attacked the nervous system causing muscle paralysis affecting breathing and possibly causing death, no longer exists in Britain because of widespread immunisation.

See separate entries for Chickenpox (page 66), German Measles (page 124), Measles (page 158), Mumps (page 166), Whooping Cough (page 214) and Tetanus Jabs (page 22).

❗ Signs and Symptoms

Most children have very minor reactions, if any at all, as a result of immunisations, and these minor side-effects are certainly not worth worrying about. They include being grumpy or crotchety, and sometimes there may be a mild fever.

There could be a local reaction such as some swelling or redness in the area where the child has been injected. If this becomes large, painful, red or very hot, seek your doctor's advice.

Immunisation timetable

The current immunisation programme is usually as follows:

3 months	immunisations against Hib, diphtheria, whooping cough, tetanus, polio
4 months	booster of above
5 months	booster of above
12–18 months	one injection against measles, mumps and rubella
3–5 years	booster injections of diphtheria and tetanus followed by a polio booster
10–14 girls	rubella immunisation if they have not received it as a baby
10–14 girls & boys	tuberculosis immunisation
school leavers	tetanus jab
15–19	polio booster

Rashes too can also develop, sometimes a few days after the immunisation has been given. It's quite normal, for instance, for children to develop a mild fever and a rash from a week to ten days after receiving the MMR immunisation (Measles, Mumps and Rubella). Some, but not many, children will experience a swelling of the face or a mild form of mumps about three weeks later.

If you are at all worried do speak to your doctor. None of the reactions from the MMR immunisations are infectious.

➕ First Aid

A mild fever can be treated with the appropriate amounts of paracetamol suspension and by following the steps under Fever (page 119) which includes keeping the child cool.

✳ A new advance: the Hib vaccine

One of the newer immunisations is Hib, which is short for Haemophilus influenza type B. The main illnesses caused by

> *A safe time to immunise*
>
> In previous times, it was thought that if the child was unwell, for example with a cold, immunisation should be delayed. Unfortunately, this often meant that the parents forgot to bring the baby back again, and not having had the proper course of injections, the infant subsequently got the illness.
>
> Consequently, since the injections are so protective and beneficial, official guidance will now usually be to immunise the child except in certain, very defined circumstances. So don't be surprised if your doctor or the professional clinic staff now advise immunisation during times that previously, with your older children perhaps, they might have suggested a delay.

this infection are a type of meningitis (the one that is most common and dangerous in children under the age of four), epiglottitis (which causes a severe swelling in the throat and difficulty in breathing), pneumonia and infections of the bones and joints. Research in the United States and Finland has demonstrated that children who have been injected against Hib infection are very well protected by the vaccine. It has already been given to 20 million children without any serious reactions to it.

New Government figures just released state that since the introduction of the vaccine in 1992, Hib has been virtually eradicated in children.

IMPALEMENT

Accidents involving impalement can be more frequent than you imagine. A person can become impaled on railings, for example, as a result of a fall from a height or from an accident when climbing.

🔴 Signs and Symptoms

An object sticking into any part of the body.

➕ First Aid

Although your first reaction, if you witness such a horrific accident, may be to try to lift the victim free, *that is the worst thing you can do*. It is not in anyone's best interest to do so until specialist help arrives. If the victim's life is not in immediate danger it is likely to be safer to make him as comfortable as possible, perhaps simply with kind words, rather than put both him and yourself in further danger if you haven't the right equipment for the job.

INDIGESTION

The stomach produces strong acid secretions which help to digest and sterilise our food. The stomach lining has a mucous coating which protects it against the acid, but the oesophagus – the gullet down which food passes from the mouth to the stomach – does not. Normally a ring of muscle – the cardiac sphincter – at the bottom end of the oesophagus acts like a trapdoor and prevents acid rising up from the stomach. When the muscle becomes lax small amounts of acid will enter the lower part of the oesophagus and cause pain and discomfort.

Probably because an attack of indigestion can be short-lived and easily treated with an antacid remedy or one of the recently released acid-blocking drugs bought from the pharmacist, three out of four indigestion sufferers never consult a doctor about it.

❗ Signs and Symptoms

Symptoms of indigestion, usually felt just below or behind the breastbone, vary from an uncomfortable feeling of fullness to nausea, pain, belching, heartburn and wind. The most common form of indigestion is heartburn – waves of burning pain behind the breastbone and sometimes a burning feeling in the throat.

➕ First Aid

As a stop gap in the absence of a professionally prepared antacid, one level teaspoonful of bicarbonate of soda dissolved in a tumblerful of water is quite effective. But it is not wise to rely on this method for long-term use since it is readily absorbed and can upset the body's delicate mineral balance.

🛇 Prevention

Smoking more than ten cigarettes a day and drinking heavily can cause indigestion. Some drugs – antibiotics, iron tablets and aspirin, for example – can cause heartburn, as can citrus fruits, chocolate, coffee and peppermint, so avoid them if you have a tendency to suffer from indigestion.

INFECTED WOUNDS

Our skin is designed to keep the inside in and the outside out, playing an important role in the immune function of the body. Yet any injury to the skin can allow germs to invade. Healing is delayed when infection sets in because blood floods to the infected wound, carrying with it the body's chemical antibodies and white cells.

This and the gunge from the local 'battle' delay the normal tissue re-construction as scar fibres are laid down prior to the tissues joining together as they heal.

This type of infection doesn't necessarily happen to a wound that's the result of an accident. Infection can set in after surgery if germs are inadvertently introduced at the time. It is to prevent this that surgeons take such care to wear sterile rubber gloves and clothing and have clean air flows through the operating theatre to keep it all as germ-free as possible.

ⓘ Signs and Symptoms

Signs that a wound is infected include more pain rather than less pain as the healing process gets underway. The wound might feel hot or look red. There could be swelling. A clear give-away is if you see yellow pus in the wound, or if the wound is oozing pus. You might also have a raised temperature with associated symptoms of hot and cold sweats, shivering and sweating.

So-called glands – not really glands at all but lymph nodes – can become swollen. These are part of the body's tissue fluid filtering system. The nodes affected will first be those that are in the direct line of drainage from the infected place.

➕ First Aid

Your first line of action will be to cover the wound with a fresh dressing and then rest the area, making sure it's raised if possible to help reduce swelling. You should see your doctor because in some cases you'll need antibiotics to clear up the infection. For a very deep and dirty wound you may need anti-tetanus injections.

INFLUENZA

Flu is caught by breathing in the virus through the germs released into the air.

❗ Signs and Symptoms

The virus attacks and inflames the lining of the nose, throat and air passages, causing symptoms similar to those of a severe cold. Joint and muscle aches and pains, headache and fever are also common, as the virus is carried by the bloodstream to other parts of the body. The worst is usually over in about a week, though an attack of flu can leave the sufferer feeling tired and depressed for some time afterwards.

➕ First Aid

The best first aid measures for influenza are rest and painkillers (paracetamol for children). Painkillers will help lower your temperature and also make you feel more comfortable. You'll need to drink plenty of watery liquids.

> ## BE CAREFUL!
>
> The complications of flu are usually due to the germs spreading to other air passages, in particular the bronchial tubes. This will make the sufferer feel particularly ill even before a cough appears. If in doubt and you are worried by the severity of the symptoms, it is wise to seek your doctor's advice.
>
> Be even more conscious of complications in someone who is very old or very young, since their antibodies and other body defences may not be so able to cope with the illness.

JELLYFISH STINGS

Swimming can be a risky business in some waters. Jellyfish don't have to be particularly big to be violent! They sting in order to catch food. So you must be extra vigilant when you are swimming while on holiday in the Mediterranean. Of course, British waters aren't without their jellyfish, particularly on the country's western coastline, and if you tread on one you will certainly know about it – the pain can be excruciating.

Signs and Symptoms

If you are stung you'll probably experience an intense stinging feeling that will be very uncomfortable. You may not feel it at the time, however, but if you develop a painful, swollen area on your body and perhaps a temperature after swimming in the sea, do consult a doctor quickly.

Sometimes allergic reactions can be provoked by jellyfish stings. Signs of this may be blisters or ulcers forming and in rare instances a severe allergic reaction can develop. See Anaphylactic Shock, page 30.

First Aid

The best treatment is to immerse the stung part in very hot – but not so hot as to scald – water. This will quickly de-activate the venom. Alcohol, vinegar, even pineapple juice or meat

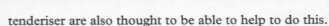

tenderiser are also thought to be able to help to do this.

If hot water isn't available, grab a handful of sand and rub over the affected area to help remove any remaining tiny hairs from the tentacles. These hairs could pierce the skin and send out more poison.

KNEE PROBLEMS

'Oh, my knees' is a cry of pain heard almost as often as 'Oh, my back'. This is hardly surprising as our knees have to bear much of our weight and are subjected to constant bending, straightening and twisting movements. The knee is one of the most complex joints in our body and, amongst sportsmen and women particularly, is the joint most commonly injured.

Three bones make up the knee joint – the ends of the thigh bone (femur) and shin bone (tibia) and the knee cap (patella). The joint is encased in a capsule lined with a membrane which secretes a lubricating fluid. It is strengthened by tough bands of tissue (ligaments), one either side of the joint and two within, which lie across each other, called the cruciate ligaments.

Also inside the joint are the two menisci – pads of tissue commonly known as the 'cartilages' – which are often involved in footballers' injuries (see also page 233). These help the knee to function efficiently. Several small fluid-filled sacs, called bursae, act as cushioning around the joint and prevent friction between the moving parts. Muscles and tendons are attached to the knee joint in various places and are responsible for supporting and moving it.

❶ Signs and Symptoms

Pain and swelling. Knees can hurt for many different reasons (see also Housemaid's Knee, page 145). Problems may occur at any age but particularly during childhood when bones and muscles are still developing and are relatively weak, and at middle age and after when bones become brittle and the muscles and tendons lax. Any part of the joint may be damaged by, for instance, accidents or over-use.

➕ First Aid

Keep the casualty off the knee if it is injured, and support the leg to lessen the pain until medical help is available. Do not administer any painkillers until the patient has been seen by a doctor as they may (rarely) need an anaesthetic for an immediate operation.

🪧 Prevention

There are a number of things you can do to protect your knees generally:

* Keep as active as possible.
* Don't sit or squat with your knees hunched up for too long and make a point of bending and straightening them fully several times a day.
* Try to avoid lifting at awkward angles or continuing any stressful activity involving the knees for a long time without a break.
* Wear suitable shoes, with cushioned, shock-absorbing insoles, for sports such as running and squash.
* Use a kneeling pad or cushion to protect your knees when necessary – while gardening, for example.

LIGHTNING STRIKES

If a person is struck by lightning they can suffer burns directly or, less commonly, as a result of clothing being set on fire.

⚠️ Signs and Symptoms

Where the lightning actually strikes and where it leaves the body as it travels to earth can be the site of a wound caused by the concentration of the electric current. The wound can be very painful since the electric charge makes the muscles go into a temporary though violent contraction. The brain, too, is subject to the shock and this is part of the reason for the violent muscle contraction that can occur. The patient may be rendered unconscious by the shock received by the brain.

> *A knock-on effect*
> Fortunately, it's surprising how few serious injuries are sustained in Britain due to lightning. But lightning can cause secondary accidents. Examples of some recently recorded accidents due to lightning include a person being bitten by a dog frightened by a storm and a woman who suffered a painful ear while using a telephone which was struck by lightning.

Lightning can also stop the heart beating as can any serious electric shock – and specialist doctors will usually want to monitor the heart after lightning has struck to confirm that it hasn't triggered an irregular heartbeat. Those who have been hit by lightning are usually knocked off their feet and suffer a terrible fright.

✚ First Aid

If the casualty is unconscious or their heart has stopped beating, carry out the procedures detailed on page 211.

If the casualty is conscious, deal with whatever symptoms are complained of – there may be none.

Take the casualty to the nearest Accident and Emergency department for their advice.

◑ Prevention

Be aware of the danger of lightning strikes. If out walking in the country when the weather changes, seek shelter on low-lying ground and never under a solitary tree which can be a good lightning conductor. On exposed ground an opened umbrella can also conduct lightning towards you, so beware!

MEASLES

Measles is very infectious and as a childhood disease it can be serious because it can lead to other complications such as ear infections, bronchitis and pneumonia. A more rare complica-

> *Did you know?*
> In the few years since an immunisation has been widely available, the incidence of measles has started to decline. From its introduction in 1989 when roughly 100,000 cases were reported in England and Wales, it has come down to 10,000 in 1992.
>
> There will no doubt be a further reduction in figures when those children who missed out just prior to its introduction are given the injection.
>
> And with each generation receiving immunisation, the people at risk will steadily decline.

tion is encephalitis (inflammation of the brain), which may lead to brain damage or convulsions. It even has the potential to kill, which it still does in large numbers in developing countries.

❗ Signs and Symptoms

A day or two before the rash of dark red spots appears on the face, behind the ears, on the arms, legs and trunk, there may be symptoms of the common cold such as inflamed, watery eyes and a high temperature. See also Immunisation Reactions, page 149.

➕ First Aid

You shouldn't take your child along to your doctor's surgery as he or she may infect others there. But do phone him to ask for advice, make the child comfortable in bed, and keep the temperature down by following the measures outlined under Fevers in Children, page 119.

MENINGITIS

Meningitis, an inflammation of the membranes surrounding the brain, is a disease feared by every parent.

There are two main types:

> *Be vigilant*
> What is urgently needed is an awareness, especially on the part of parents, of the danger signs. If your child shows any of the suspicious symptoms, remember – consult a doctor without delay no matter what time of night or day. If meningitis is suspected hospitalisation will be necessary.

* viral meningitis, which is more common, usually less severe and cannot be helped by antibiotic treatment
* bacterial meningitis, which is generally more serious, requiring urgent treatment with antibiotics

The most common serious form of bacterial meningitis to affect babies, especially in the first year of life, is due to Hib – Haemophilus influenza B. There is now an injection against this so the number of babies affected is diminishing rapidly. It was introduced in 1992, and in only two years the notified cases of Hib were down by an astonishing 92%. (See also page 150.)

Meningitis is most often found in children and can cause brain damage, gangrene, deafness and even death. It is infectious, strikes randomly and there are very few precautions you can take against it. But although meningitis is a potentially fatal disease, many, if not most, of the people who get it make a complete recovery – given time.

❗ Signs and Symptoms

The most important weapon in fighting meningitis is speed. The early and common symptoms may be no more than a headache, raised temperature and perhaps some sickness.

➕ First Aid

If you suspect that these symptoms are somehow more worrying or different, act immediately before the more obvious symptoms – severe malaise, strong dislike of light (photophobia), drowsiness, neck stiffness and a red or pinkish rash –

become apparent. When someone has meningitis, especially bacterial meningitis, the membranes covering the brain and central nervous system are inflamed and any movement of the neck causes severe pain. Consequently, the neck muscles often go into a reflex spasm to prevent movement and so protect the sufferer from further pain.

MIGRAINE

Migraine is usually a very severe headache that can vary in duration and intensity from person to person. See also Headaches, page 133.

❗ Signs and Symptoms

What makes migraine more than 'just a headache'? The pain is usually one sided, and there can be symptoms such as loss of appetite, nausea or vomiting. Some sufferers will have migraine with an aura – that is, a migraine which is preceded, twenty to thirty minutes before the headache itself, by warning symptoms, which may include flashing lights before the eyes, shimmering or double vision, slurred speech, numbness and giddiness. These symptoms are probably due to a sudden constriction in some of the blood vessels in the brain. The headache comes on as these vessels then expand and the blood surges through, leading to the characteristic throbbing headache.

➕ First Aid

Anti-inflammatory medicines such as aspirin and ibuprofen can prevent the release of prostaglandin and are recommended for migraine, although paracetamol can help ease the pain of a headache, too.

Any medicines should be taken at the first sign of an attack, so always keep them handy if you are a migraine sufferer. It usually helps to rest quietly in a darkened room during the early stages.

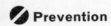 **Prevention**

Irregular meals, dieting or a long lie-in can provoke a migraine, probably because of the drop in the body's blood sugar. A few biscuits or a sweet drink may be enough to stave off a full attack.

It's extremely important to make sure you always eat properly and pay attention to your diet. If you think you'll have to go a long time without a proper meal, keep an emergency ration of some sort with you.

MISCARRIAGE

Anyone who has experienced a miscarriage – the loss of a pregnancy before the twenty-eighth week – will know that it is distressing however early it occurs.

Signs and Symptoms

When you are pregnant, vaginal bleeding accompanied by back pain or cramping pains in the lower abdomen can be a warning sign of a miscarriage and you must get in touch with your doctor as soon as possible. Sometimes in early pregnancy there can be a spotting of blood around the time a menstrual period would normally be due. Other causes are a vaginal infection or an erosion on the cervix.

In later pregnancy vaginal bleeding can be a sign that:

* labour is beginning
* the placenta is becoming separated from the womb's wall
* the placenta is in a low position covering the entrance to the womb
* there are defects in the cervix

So bleeding at any stage of pregnancy needs medical attention and advice.

162

Did you know?
Studies show that many miscarriages occur so early on that the woman has not even missed a period or realised she is pregnant, but at least one in six confirmed pregnancies end in miscarriage too. It is also quite common to have two or three consecutive miscarriages – the cause in each case may be different or unknown – but more than half of women who miscarry in this way will then go on to have a normal healthy baby without any treatment at all.

➕ First Aid

If you are beginning to lose blood you should wear a maternity sanitary pad. Your doctor may advise hospital admission, particularly if the blood loss is severe. If a miscarriage is confirmed, you will probably be given a D&C (dilation and curettage) operation to remove the womb's contents.

There is no definite evidence that rest in bed prevents a threatened miscarriage although it may help to relieve anxiety and make you feel you are doing all you can. Consequently it is still often advised.

✳ Afterwards

Well-meaning people may say, 'Never mind, you can always try again,' but that is no real consolation because, for you, that particular baby cannot be replaced.

Perhaps you felt to blame in case something you did or did not do caused the miscarriage (though this is most unlikely). It may help to know that miscarriage, also known by doctors as abortion whether it occurs unexpectedly (spontaneous abortion) or deliberately (therapeutic abortion) is very common indeed, possibly three out of four conceptions end in this way.

Following a miscarriage, a time of grieving is usually important for the mother and also the father. It should help, if possible, to know the sex of the baby, perhaps to see it, and to talk to an understanding person, preferably one who has been through the same experience.

> *Ectopic pregnancy*
> Any bleeding in pregnancy needs to be discussed with your doctor. Sometimes bleeding accompanied by pain or a sudden and severe abdominal pain during the first few weeks of pregnancy could be signs of an ectopic pregnancy which will need *immediate* medical treatment. This occurs when a fertilised egg develops outside the womb, usually in one of the fallopian tubes.

Individual needs and reactions will vary greatly depending on the circumstances. Opinions differ as to whether it is best to wait about three months before trying to become pregnant again to allow for physical and emotional adjustment or to try again straight away. Either way, the chances of a successful outcome next time are high.

✳ Causes of miscarriage

It is understandable after a miscarriage to ask why it should be you. It's understandable, too, to look for an explanation. Many occur because something goes wrong at a very early stage in the development of the foetus or the placenta – not really surprising when one realises what a complex process this is. Abnormalities occurring in the baby's genetic make-up or in its developing heart or nervous system are other likely causes. Some drugs or an infection, such as German measles and heavy drinking or smoking, may cause abnormalities in the foetus and lead to miscarriage. Fibroids or polyps (benign growths) which protrude into the womb, or an IUD left in place during pregnancy, are among other possible causes. Often, however, particularly if miscarriage occurs in the first three months of pregnancy, the cause cannot be pinpointed.

In the second three months, miscarriage is much less common and the cause is often apparent and treatable – for example, an incompetent cervix, which also accounts for many recurrent miscarriages. The cervix (neck of the womb) may have been damaged during an operation or by a previous birth, especially if the baby was large. Occasionally it is just naturally lax.

Normally, during pregnancy the cervical hole, which is the

entrance to the womb, remains tightly closed until contractions in the first stage of labour dilate it to allow the baby through. With an incompetent cervix the hole is already slightly open and pressure on it as the baby grows larger increases the gap until the baby almost 'falls out'. Once the problem has been diagnosed the gynaecologist can insert a special stitch around the cervix for support – usually done about the fourteenth week of pregnancy – which is removed as the delivery date approaches.

Some specialists believe that a lack of the hormone progesterone may cause repeated miscarriages and will give, for example, progesterone pessaries (also called suppositories) to counteract this. In some women recurrent miscarriage may be due to their body's 'rejection' of the foetus – similar to the rejection that can follow a kidney transplant.

Research into possible solutions continues.

Prevention

Most women who have had one or more miscarriages will want to do all they can to avoid another. It will help not to smoke or drink alcohol, to avoid all non-essential medicines and to eat a good varied diet, even before conception.

If you have experienced some bleeding it is probably wise to avoid intercourse for two weeks afterwards as orgasm causes contractions in the womb and might add to the risks. The bleeding will come from the mother and not the baby and the baby will not therefore be damaged if the pregnancy is able to continue.

MOSQUITO BITES

See Gnat Bites, page 126.

MOUTH ULCERS

Mouth ulcers can cause pain in the mouth on the inside of the cheeks as well as on the gums.

❗ Signs and Symptoms

The first sign of a mouth ulcer will be pain coming from the gum or inside of the cheek. When you look inside your mouth you will probably find a mouth ulcer, called an aphthous ulcer, a small lesion which has a grey base and a slightly raised yellowish edge, tinged with a narrow, inflamed border.

Symptoms can appear before the ulcer itself. The mouth can become over-sensitive or there will be a burning or tingling sensation.

➕ First Aid

Mouth ulcers usually clear up within a few days but can take over a week to disappear. In most cases, no treatment is needed, but if the ulcer is particularly painful, an antiseptic mouthwash or pastilles containing antiseptics and local anaesthetics can ease soreness.

If ulcers do persist or occur frequently it may be wise to consult your doctor to check that there is no underlying cause.

MUMPS

Mumps can be a nasty disease.

The child is infectious for a week before symptoms develop and for a week after, and the total incubation period is about eighteen days. The disease can be avoided if you have your child immunised (see Immunisation Reactions, page 149).

Before puberty complications are uncommon. After puberty mumps oophoritis in a woman (inflammation of the ovaries) can cause abdominal pain but rarely anything worse. More common is orchiditis in a man (inflammation of the testes). This can be both painful and cause lasting damage since the outer capsule of the testicle is tough and unelastic. Any swelling can't expand outwards so the pressure builds up and can destroy the internal lining tissue – replacing it subsequently with non-functional scar tissue. If this happens to both testes sterility can ensue – though fortunately this is rare.

Mumps meningitis, a potentially serious inflammation of the brain's covering, can occur, though it is not common and total recovery is usual.

❗ Signs and Symptoms

Symptoms are swelling in the angle behind the jaw because the salivary glands are inflamed, a high temperature, headache and loss of appetite. Unlike many other childhood diseases, mumps doesn't cause a rash.

✱ First Aid

The pain and fever may be treated with paracetamol suspension and the patient may need a liquid diet, as eating can sometimes prove very painful.

A painful testicle can be greatly relieved when supported by a suspensory bandage available from the pharmacist.

NECK PAIN

Neck pain and stiffness are very common, particularly as we get older. The neck is made up of seven cervical vertebrae – bones which are part of the spinal column or backbone – with cushioning discs in between, strengthened on either side by many muscles and ligaments. These normally allow the neck to move easily and help to support the weight of the head as it pivots on the topmost, Atlas vertebra. The cervical vertebrae and the rest of the backbone protect the spinal cord, from which nerves branch out through openings in the vertebrae to the neck and arms and other parts of the body.

With the constant movements of the head and neck it is no wonder that wear and tear, known as cervical spondylosis, occurs in time. In fact, it begins around the age of twenty-five! This accounts for most neck stiffness, though will not necessarily cause pain as well.

The discs between the vertebrae also harden with age and lose their shock-absorbing effect, while bony outgrowths, called osteophytes, develop around their edges.

🛈 Signs and Symptoms

Osteophytes pressing on a nerve can lead to pain in the neck and numbness, tingling or weakness in the shoulders or arms, depending on which nerve is affected. Wear and tear can also damage the lining of the neck joints and cause osteoarthritic pain.

Neck pain can be a symptom of other forms of arthritis such as rheumatoid arthritis and ankylosing spondylitis and, more rarely, of other conditions – meningitis and poliomyelitis, for instance. Pain in the neck may also be caused by overstretching the ligaments and tendons as they try to compensate for neck stiffness elsewhere.

Sometimes a stiff, painful neck develops for no apparent reason only to disappear after a few days. The clicking and grating sounds – known as crepitus – that we can often hear as we move our head are due to roughened bony surfaces rubbing against each other and are not usually harmful.

➕ First Aid

Nine out of ten times, neck pain will get better without a doctor's treatment. Muscles surrounding a painful area often go into spasm to try to protect it – although this can also add to the pain. This cycle may be broken by taking painkillers, such as aspirin or ibuprofen, regularly for a few days to relieve the pain and allow the muscle spasm to subside. Warmth (a covered and comfortably hot water bottle on the neck, for instance) will also help to relax tense muscles and massage can be very soothing, at least temporarily.

If pain is persistent your doctor may advise you to wear a special neck collar for a while. This, by restricting movement, allows the damaged joints to rest and can be very effective. Traction – stretching of the neck – may be suggested if there appears to be nerve pressure but this must only be done by a doctor, physiotherapist or other qualified professional. Manipulation by a registered osteopath or chiropractor can also be helpful.

Prevention

Neck pain can be caused by sleeping with too many pillows, sitting for a long time at a low desk with your head bent down, looking upwards for too long – while painting a ceiling, for example – and any repetitive movement of the arm or shoulder. Being aware of how you carry out everyday tasks and making them as comfortable as possible can help you avoid neck pain. A whiplash injury (see page 213) from a car accident is another common cause which can often be prevented by using headrests.

> **BE CAREFUL!**
>
> If your neck pain is severe and getting worse, or if you have any numbness or 'pins and needles', do consult a doctor.

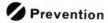

NOSE BLEEDS

There's not always an obvious or apparent reason for a nose bleed. The bleeding can vary from a small spot of blood to a mini flood. When we lose blood, there often appears to be much more of it than there actually is. It's as if nature has given us an inbuilt defence mechanism – we see blood in all its startling redness and we know that we must do something about it quickly.

In children and young adults, the most common cause of a nose bleed is inflammation of an area on the lining of the partition of the nose – the septum. This condition causes the area – known as Little's area – to look red on examination and, if touched, it will bleed easily. Most nose bleeds that occur due to inflammation of Little's area can be stopped by the measures mentioned below.

Signs and Symptoms

Nose bleeds most often occur in young people, especially teenagers. Usually the bleeding will make a mess of half a dozen handkerchiefs and that will be the end of it. But when the blood flow doesn't stop and the sufferer dabs at the nose anxiously, any clot starting to form will be knocked off. This, of course, prevents nature from curing the problem.

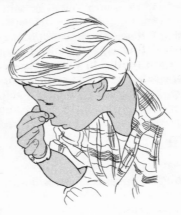

✚ First Aid

Even large arteries in the body, if damaged through an injury, will stop bleeding eventually if firm pressure is applied. So it may help you to stay calm if you remind yourself that the blood vessels in the nose are really very small indeed, so pinching the lower part of the nose for about ten minutes should be enough to stop the bleeding. It may also help to sit down while you are doing this, especially if you lean forward slightly over a

---

Did you know?

I know people sometimes think that high blood pressure causes nose bleeds. But this is rarely so – although in later middle age and beyond, blood pressure is more likely to be on the high side and, coupled with a 'hardening of the arteries', continual nose bleeds can be potentially more serious.

In rare instances, frequent nose bleeds may be due to a blood disorder which will need medical attention. Your doctor may want to take a sample of blood from an arm to send for tests. However, the chances of you having any blood disorder are extremely remote.

bowl, so blood can trickle out of the mouth if it collects there.

If the frequency of your nose bleeds becomes a real worry to you, then do go to your doctor. Usually your GP or a specialist will cauterise the offending blood vessels, which are to be found inside the nostrils on the wall of the septum.

But, once in a while, elderly sufferers (and occasionally younger people) will find that the bleeding just won't stop, whatever methods are tried. On these rare occasions, an ear, nose and throat specialist will need to perform an operation to 'tie off' a branch of the arterial blood supply to the nose.

Once the artery is closed off, the body compensates for its loss by opening up other small vessels from nearby arteries, so that blood still gets through to the nasal tissues.

NOSES, FOREIGN OBJECT IN

❗ Signs and Symptoms

A discharge – often blood-stained, yellow or green mucus – may be the first sign that there's anything wrong, or the child may complain of discomfort in the nose if something like a pea or a button, for example, has been pushed into the nostrils.

➕ First Aid

Don't try to dislodge the object yourself because you may cause further damage.

An experienced ENT surgeon may be able to remove the object without the need for a general anaesthetic, though not if the child is too terrified to keep still, or, understandably, is crying his head off. The extra nasal liquid present and the forced expirations that crying causes may produce the offending object without more ado.

PALPITATIONS

Palpitations are very common and for most people it's simply a case of being suddenly and unusually aware of their heart beating, noticed most especially in bed at night.

ⓘ Signs and Symptoms

The beating may be unusually fast, strong, fluttering or just quicker than usual.

Once a person becomes aware of their heart beating (for whatever harmless reason), they may feel anxious. This causes adrenaline to be released in the body, which then makes the heart beat faster and more forcibly – and firmly fixes in the person's mind the idea that something is wrong with them.

➕ First Aid

A doctor's reassurance is often enough on its own to 'cure' these common palpitations. When it isn't then relaxation techniques may also need to be practised. Concentrating on deep, steady breathing can calm the nerves and hence the palpitations.

✳ Is there something wrong?

Occasionally, palpitations can be a sign that something is physically wrong. In some rare instances it's not a question of the individual being unusually aware of their heartbeat, but of the heartbeat itself being unusual.

This kind of palpitation is known by doctors as an arrhythmia – an abnormal beating of the heart, either in rhythm or in force, or quite often both. The two most common kinds are:

* ectopic beats, when an extra beat of the heart occurs too rapidly after the previous one and an abnormally long pause then follows it
* paroxysmal – or re-entrant – tachycardia, when the heart's natural pace-maker is blanked out by the heart's electrical conduction mechanism. This rapidly re-excites the heart's muscle which therefore keeps beating very rapidly – right out of the blue.

With ectopic beats, the heart's normal triggering mechanism is interrupted by an extra trigger. It's a bit like the engine of a car ticking over normally and then suddenly being interrupted by an extra spark plug, which causes an upset in the normal rhythm.

Re-entrant tachycardia is due to extra 'wiring' in the heart causing the part of the heart that's active to excite another part of the heart that's resting. This sets up a cycle of continuous fast and regular or irregular heartbeating.

For every person who experiences these definite changes in heartbeat rhythm, however, there will be vast numbers who suffer from palpitations even though their heart is beating normally.

So if you are at all worried, do see your doctor. He will be able to make the correct diagnosis and refer you to a specialist, if necessary.

PANIC ATTACKS AND HYPERVENTILATION

Sometimes otherwise fit and healthy people suffer waves of light-headedness which make them feel as if they are going to faint or be sick (though they rarely do either). When these attacks come on out of the blue they are likely to be a mild form of panic attack. More severe attacks involve palpitations, sensations of heaviness in the chest, sweaty palms and so on.

Hyperventilation – overbreathing – may also occur. The sufferer may experience a tingling sensation around the mouth, cramp in his hands and may soon be covered in very small red spots, called petechiae.

➕ First Aid

Panic attacks can be overcome when you appreciate what they are – simply a series of symptoms that can't hurt you. Try this relaxation technique. Sit down if you can and let your shoulders and jaw relax while taking slow and deep breaths. Concentrate on doing this until the moment passes. Also tell yourself that you are not going to faint.

If this doesn't help go to your doctor for advice. In some cases tablets called beta-blockers may be prescribed which can prevent your heart racing and will have a mildly tranquillising effect.

If the sufferer is hyperventilating, encourage them to re-breath their own expired air from a paper (not plastic) bag, opened and held loosely over their nose and mouth. This soon corrects the deficiency of carbon dioxide in their blood and the symptoms subside.

PENIS, FOREIGN OBJECT IN

Now and then small children have been known to push small beads or similar objects into the foreskin, or more rarely into the urine hole (the urethra) of the penis, which can cause an infection if left there.

❶ Signs and Symptoms

The first you might know of such an accident is when you notice a discharge from the child's penis. The same accident happens with girls pushing small objects into their vagina which, too, can cause infection. Warning signs of such an infection could be a greyish-yellow or greenish vaginal discharge.

➕ First Aid

This type of emergency needs medical attention without delay.

PERFORATED EARDRUM

Any injury to the ear can cause an eardrum to be perforated – sticking a cotton bud into the ear, being hit on the side of the head, even the force of an explosion. The force of a sudden bang on the ear, or a loud noise, can cause great differences in pressure inside the ear which can result in damage, such as a hole in the ear drum.

❶ Signs and Symptoms

Blood coming from the inside of the ear is a sign that the eardrum is perforated. Other less obvious warning signs are:

* deafness in the ear following an injury, or an infection
* pain which is suddenly relieved

* a discharge which eases the pain once you notice it forming
* a ringing in the ears which is known as tinnitus

➕ First Aid

On no account treat this type of injury at home. You must get the person to the nearest Accident and Emergency department with their head leaning to one side in order to let blood flow out rather than collect in the ear.

PERIOD PAIN

In most cases painful periods are not a sign of ill health, but women who suddenly develop them should go to see their doctor, so that the cause can be treated appropriately. Sufferers of primary dysmenorrhoea (the kind of pain suffered by younger women) sometimes have more of a chemical called prostaglandin in their menstrual flow than most women. The production of an egg, or ovum, in the middle of the month triggers the release of this excess prostaglandin, which sends pain signals to the brain – so when a woman doesn't ovulate she usually doesn't experience pain. That's why many women who suffer from painful periods are advised to take the contraceptive pill, which generally works by preventing ovulation – this is a relatively straightforward way to bring relief.

❗ Signs and Symptoms

A cramp-like pain as soon as the period starts, or a dull ache in the abdomen and back.

➕ First Aid

Painkillers can help you cope with period pain. An anti-inflammatory one called ibuprofen can inhibit the production of prostaglandin, which is why it can be so effective in relieving symptoms. Aspirin has the same effect. They can both be purchased from your pharmacy.

Hot baths can also be soothing for period pain. Heat in the

form of a hot water bottle can help reduce muscle spasm, as can brisk exercise such as cycling, swimming and fast walking.

PILES

Doctors believe that at least half the people in Britain suffer from piles at some time in their life, although many are too embarrassed to seek advice. Piles (also known as haemorrhoids) are engorged veins – varicose veins that may feel rather like soft, spongy grapes.

❗ Signs and Symptoms

Piles are found in and around the lower rectum and anal canal at the very lowest end of the bowel, in a pad of tissue that is not unlike the lips of the mouth. You may notice itching, small spots of fresh, red blood on the toilet paper after bowel movement, or a discharge of mucus from the anus.

You are more likely to suffer from piles as you get older (especially if you are overweight), although younger people can suffer too.

➕ First Aid

For very painful external piles, such as a protruding pile which has become strangulated after being gripped by the tight muscular band (sphincter) at the exit to the anus, rest in bed with the foot of the bed raised. An ice pack applied to the pile should relieve pain. If the blood inside the pile then clots, it will, in time, drop off – providing nature's cure.

For less severe piles, you can try some suppositories and/or ointments recommended by your pharmacist and follow their instructions. These mainly contain local anaesthetics to ease irritation and astringents to help dry up piles and relieve inflammation.

For piles that recur and become troublesome you should seek your doctor's advice because specialist treatment may be needed, such as injection treatment to shrink the piles or cryosurgery to 'freeze' the veins.

BE CAREFUL!

Any bleeding after a bowel movement should be checked by your doctor to establish that it is caused by haemorrhoids and not any other condition.

Prevention

Less severe piles can often be cured completely by avoiding constipation and straining. This means eating plenty of high-fibre foods – fresh fruit and vegetables, wholemeal bread and bran cereals, for instance. Try also to cut down on salt and have plenty of watery or fruit drinks. This type of diet should keep your motions regular, well-formed and effortless. Laxatives are usually only advisable as a short-term measure.

Fact not fiction

There are many old wives' tales about the causes of piles. Despite popular belief, you do not get them by sitting on cold walls or floors nor hot radiators. Perhaps surprisingly, active sportsmen and women are prone to piles and, like varicose veins, they are a particular hazard of pregnancy. The weight of the developing baby can put pressure on the rectal veins, causing them to enlarge as the normal flow of blood is prevented. Fortunately, these piles usually subside after the baby's birth and treatment meanwhile can relieve the discomfort.

Some medicines, such as codeine and iron tablets, if taken regularly, can be constipating and so predispose to piles. However, chronic constipation, with the straining and increased pressure on the veins this brings, is one of the most common likely causes; as is a lack of fibre in the diet over many years.

PULLED MUSCLES

See Strains, Sprains and Pulled Muscles, page 193.

PUNCTURE WOUNDS

Puncture wounds caused, for example, when a nail goes into the palm of your hand while doing some home repairs need careful attention. In extreme cases, an infection resulting from such an injury can interfere with the movement of the fingers.

🚫 Signs and Symptoms

If a nail, or some other sharp object, penetrates the tough fibres just below the skin of the palm it can carry an infection that will result in inflammation behind that sheet of fibres. This will cause pain and tenderness and, in the long term, scar tissue could form which will restrict the function of the fingers.

➕ First Aid

The chances of getting a general infection from such a perforating injury are quite high, so this is why you'll sometimes be advised to take antibiotics. There is also the risk of tetanus (see page 22). If you suffer a puncture wound you do need to see your doctor or for more serious wounds go to your nearest hospital Accident and Emergency department.

If in pain, take some of your usual painkilling tablets in the meantime. If it is bleeding, cover with a clean cloth and apply pressure after letting some blood – about three teaspoons full – run out of the wound. This carries away many if not most of the germs that got in!

RAPE

When a woman has been raped or sexually assaulted she will need understanding, sympathy and tender care. Your first reaction will perhaps be to offer her a drink but this really isn't the best course of action as far as the police are concerned. A victim of rape, or other form of sexual abuse, will immediately want to have a bath, or a wash to scrub away the brutal invasion of her body but, understandable as this may be, it mustn't be done. Having a drink, washing or even going to the loo could tamper with vital forensic evidence, such as semen, blood or samples of hair. The victim should be urged to contact the police as soon as possible.

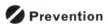 Prevention

Don't put yourself in jeopardy. Avoid unlit short cuts and travelling alone at night. Make sure you check the identification of all unknown callers at your door. Enrol in a self-awareness/defence class so that you can both assess likely dangerous situations and know what to do if you find yourself in one.

RASHES

When do you need to worry about a rash in a child? The answer has to be when it is unusual, severe, occurs in association with other symptoms like a fever or a headache or it is a mild one that persists enough to worry you.

SCRATCHES

Scratches usually pass off without incident unless germs are introduced and they become infected.

✚ First Aid

Clean the scratch thoroughly with cold running water if possible and follow the measures outlined for cuts and lacerations (page 84).

Did you know?
A scratch from a cat can occasionally carry a virus which can make the sufferer's lymph nodes (commonly called glands) enlarge either body wide or locally. It's called cat scratch syndrome and it usually gets better on its own though it must be reported to the doctor to be sure of the diagnosis.

SHOCK

All manner of things can trigger a state of shock. The body's reactions to a physical injury, often called a surgical shock (when a large amount of blood may be lost) and to an emotional shock (a severe fright) are remarkably similar. What happens is this. The blood pressure drops suddenly and drastically so the person passes out and falls to the floor if they were standing, or goes cold, clammy, has a very weak pulse and may become unconscious if they are lying flat.

❗ Signs and Symptoms

Signs that a person is in shock are a rapid but weak pulse, sweating, a pale face, trembling, quick light breathing, clammy skin and feeling cold. Secondary reactions include weakness, dizziness, vomiting or feeling very thirsty.

➕ First Aid

If after any accident a person looks pale and unwell and appears to be suffering from symptoms of shock, send for emergency help at once. While you are waiting for it to arrive you must make them lie down with their feet raised on cushions, books, or whatever is available. This is particularly useful if a lot of blood has been lost as it sends more blood to the brain. But don't do this if you think the casualty has a head injury or a broken leg. Try not to move the casualty more than you need to. Warm the person by covering them up to conserve their body heat, but don't apply any heat sources as this can burn the skin and tissues due to the

Delayed shock
Delayed shock is the term used when the symptoms don't start until some time after the accident, injury or fright. It can take many forms but the usual signs are fits of crying, shaking or depression. If severe it may become Post Traumatic Stress Syndrome, needing specialist psychological or psychiatric help.

sluggish peripheral blood supply and the now slow reflexes of the sufferer.

Reassurance helps a great deal when a person is in shock. Anxiety or sensations of panic can only serve to make the physical symptoms of shock even worse. Treat any other problems such as cuts and bleeding which may be present.

> **BE CAREFUL!**
>
> Shock can be serious. When it's severe or not treated in time, death can ensue. Occasionally the shock can result in a fatality even though the injury may have been relatively minor.

SICKNESS IN BABIES AND CHILDREN

How does a mother know if her baby or child is really sick and there is cause for genuine panic? Firstly, worry has to be your guide. If you consider that your baby or child is unwell, even if there aren't any obvious symptoms, you should contact your doctor for advice.

Signs and Symptoms

Any of the following warning signs need urgent medical attention:

* if a child has a fit or turns blue or is very pale
* quick, difficult breathing or breathing that sounds like grunting
* if a baby or child is very hard to wake or is unusually drowsy
* if a child doesn't seem to be able to recognise people he or she knows well

You should seek a doctor's advice immediately if after a fall or other accident your child:

* is unconscious
* is vomiting

* feeling drowsy
* if there's any blood coming from the ears
* if he or she has lost a lot of blood
* seems to be in pain internally, or complains of severe pain anywhere

Symptoms that signify your baby or child is unwell and needs to see a doctor include:

* a deep cough accompanied by noisy breathing
* any unusual bouts of crying which can signify pain or discomfort
* if he or she refuses feeds several times
* any repeated vomiting
* diarrhoea
* a child who is very hot, very cold or floppy

BE CAREFUL!

Even if you have spoken to or consulted your doctor, but a baby or child does not seem to be improving, or is definitely getting worse, you must contact your doctor again.

SICKNESS IN THE ELDERLY

The illnesses that generally and suddenly affect elderly people include the common cold, influenza, bronchitis, pleurisy, pneumonia and urinary tract infections.

The very old are especially at risk from complications as a result of a cold or similar infection. They should be watched carefully in case their symptoms worsen. The ageing immune (disease-fighting) system and other bodily defences are less effective at combating infection and the elderly are particularly vulnerable.

! Signs and Symptoms

So how will you know when to call a doctor? The following symptoms need medical attention:

* coughing up green, as opposed to clear, sputum (a sure sign that a secondary bacterial infection has developed and antibiotics may then be needed)
* a very bad cough
* streaks of blood in the sputum
* breathlessness, wheezing
* 'tightness' or pain in the chest
* blueness around the lips

It is also wise to consult a doctor if the patient's temperature, pulse and breathing rate rise and he or she seems generally unwell. In fact, real concern is a good criterion for asking a doctor's opinion in any circumstances – if only for reassurance – and this applies as much to symptoms associated with the 'common cold' as to anything else.

* Bronchitis and pneumonia

Most attacks of bronchitis follow an infection of the lining membranes in the nose, throat or sinuses – what doctors call an upper respiratory infection. This is because once a cold, influenza or a respiratory virus invades the nose and upper membranes, it can so easily extend its invasion downwards and affect the main breathing tubes. These airways are called the bronchi.

Indeed, if the germ is a particularly virulent one, or if the sufferer's defences are low, then it can spread down into the smaller tubes, the bronchioles, often causing bronchiolitis. Sometimes it even infects the final breathing membrane, when

---

How you can help – the flu vaccine
One way to help prevent complications such as pneumonia and pleurisy is to make sure an elderly person is offered a flu vaccination each year (the best time is in the autumn). Immunisation against flu is becoming increasingly widespread in Britain. A vaccination given in the autumn provides about 70 per cent protection and lasts about a year. Most doctors believe it's worthwhile for the vulnerable groups because flu can be a serious illness for them.

> *Confusion in the elderly*
> I'm often asked whether episodes of confusion in the elderly can be due to illness. Yes, chest infections or urinary tract infections can cause some elderly people to become confused. In the case of pneumonia, the person may suddenly become confused but have only minor chest symptoms, so be on the look out for this and call the doctor without delay if you are concerned.

it causes pneumonia. At that stage, because there is so much of that membrane (if spread out it could cover several table-tennis tables), the infection makes a real assault upon the body's defences. That's why pneumonia, especially, is treated with antibiotics. Before these were available, many attacks of pneumonia ended in tragedy.

✳ Pleurisy

Pleurisy can develop as a complication of pneumonia.

Symptoms will include a sharp pain on breathing in, a high temperature, general malaise and a cough. There are two types of pleurisy, dry or wet. In dry pleurisy, the pleura (two delicate membranes separating the lungs from the chest wall) become inflamed. In wet pleurisy more fluid is produced than is needed, secreted by the inflamed membranes and filling up the space between them. Pleurisy can be serious and will need treatment with antibiotics.

✳ Urinary tract infections

Urinary tract infections commonly affect the elderly. Symptoms will include frequency in passing urine, incontinence, offensive smelling urine and pain when passing it. This type of infection will need to be checked by a doctor as it may require treatment with an antibiotic. As well as antibiotics the elderly person will also need to drink plenty.

These infections can cause acute confusion in the elderly, and when this is the case the patient may fail to mention the symptoms. If confusion has come on very suddenly a doctor will often suspect, and test for, urinary tract infections.

SNAKE BITES

Snake bites in Britain are unlikely to be too serious – the adder is our only venomous snake.

🛇 Signs and Symptoms

The sufferer will complain of great pain. There may be obvious pierce marks where the snake has bitten them.

➕ First Aid

Common first aid measures such as sucking the wound or making an incision with a razor blade to squeeze out the venom can do more harm than good. It's best just to immobilise the bitten limb, by bandaging it to the body or by using a sling, and take the person straight to hospital.

SOLVENT ABUSE (Glue Sniffing)

Solvent abuse is nothing new – it was first reported in this country in the sixties. Nor is it an epidemic. In fact, recent surveys showed that while 97 per cent of school-aged children were aware of glue sniffing, only 8 per cent had ever tried it.

Solvent abuse isn't confined to any particular social class or area. But the majority of those involved are teenagers in the fourteen to seventeen age group, who are out for kicks or to impress their friends, or like the attraction of shocking their parents. It is a habit that is usually picked up in the playground by a group of children, and is generally abandoned as quickly as any other craze.

Now, thanks to organisations like Re-Solv and the Institute for the Study of Drug Dependence (ISDD), there is a growing network of counselling agencies, helplines and drug units able to deal with all aspects of solvent abuse.

🛇 Signs and Symptoms

It can sometimes be difficult to know whether a young person has been sniffing solvents. Although solvent sniffing is not illegal, they are not very likely to admit to you that they have been trying to get 'high' with aerosol spray, cigarette lighter fuel, dry-cleaning fluids, paint and paint thinners, solvent-containing correcting fluids such as Tipp-Ex (although you can now buy a solvent-free Tipp-Ex), even petrol. It's not just glue that can be sniffed!

Symptoms to look out for in a persistent solvent abuser include:

* running eyes and nose
* a rash around the nose
* poor muscle control
* loss of appetite and weight loss
* mood swings
* frequent headaches and sore throats

Not all sniffing incidents can result in unconsciousness.

A one-off experiment may result in the child behaving as if he or she were drunk. Solvent abuse can make a child more reckless than normal. 'Mild' effects can include dizziness, confusion, lethargy, loss of attention and nausea.

✚ First Aid

If you find your child drowsy or unconscious, and you suspect he or she may have been sniffing solvents, you must act speedily to ensure that they are surrounded by plenty of fresh air. Open doors and windows quickly. The casualty needs to be turned on to his or her side in the recovery position (see page 18). If you can get someone to dial 999 while you are doing this, all the better. If not, put the casualty into the recovery position first, then rush to the phone.

If there is evidence nearby of what the person has been sniffing collect it up, containers, tablets, anything that is suspect and give it to the ambulance crew. Many parents fail to realise that substances may be sniffed in a variety of ways, from bags such as crisp packets to coatsleeves.

You must stay with the child until the effects have worn off.

It is not wise to get angry and approach them in a threatening way. There have been instances when children have exerted themselves suddenly in response, often running away, which

> *Glue-sniffing – some facts*
> There are more than one hundred deaths each year from solvent sniffing, and most of these deaths are among teenagers. Unlike harder drugs, or even cigarettes, solvent abuse is rarely addictive, apart from a psychological dependence, though this can still prove difficult to break. Research shows that the majority of children who experiment with sniffing rapidly give it up, their attention diverted by girl or boyfriends, sport or other interests.
>
> There are, for course, potential risks to health involved in solvent abuse. Users can suffer heart or lung problems and possible damage to the liver and kidneys. But, so far, there is no conclusive proof of any long-term health problems in children after they stop abusing solvents. The biggest danger is that a former long-term user may become a heavy drinker or smoker to fill the void.

has resulted in tragedy. The lack of oxygen and the circulation of toxins, both caused by the sniffing, have put the heart under strain and a sudden exertion has proved the final straw.

Whatever you want to say or do, wait until you both feel better and the atmosphere is much calmer.

SORE THROAT

The exact cause of a sore throat can only be established as other symptoms develop. And there are many possible causes – it may be due to a virus and mean the start of a cold or flu. It is also one of the first signs of German measles or pharyngitis and tonsillitis, which may need antibiotics. So if sore throat symptoms persist, consult your doctor.

❗ Signs and Symptoms

Pain. A sore throat is an infection making the throat red and sore, most often due to a viral infection which clears up by itself after three or four days.

A sore throat can also be caused by a bacterium called the

streptococcus. One branch of this germ family has recently been associated with a very rare condition called necrotising fasciitis. When the germs are able to become established in the fascia (or plane just below the skin) – after an operation or injury, for example – they can release toxins which destroy the tissues and cause a severe illness in the sufferer. Fortunately it is very rare, doesn't seem to be on the increase and should not be a cause for general anxiety or fear.

✚ First Aid

Pain can be relieved by taking soluble aspirin or your preferred painkiller (paracetamol for children). Avoid smoking if your throat is very sore. Try gargling with a teaspoonful of salt in a tumbler of warm water or a mixture of lemon juice and honey in warm water. These can be great soothers. As can the gargles or pastilles the pharmacist may suggest.

SPINAL INJURY

Spinal injuries are serious because the spinal cord carrying the nerves controlling several of the body's functions could be injured, or further damaged if you try to move the patient. A fractured spine will eventually heal and may cause little subsequent disability if the spinal cord is intact. If the spinal cord is damaged there could be permanent paralysis of the legs, or arms and legs.

❗ Signs and Symptoms

Warning signs include a numb or paralysed leg or trunk. There may also be pain in any part of the spine if movement is attempted or difficulty in breathing or pain when passing urine.

✚ First Aid

If you suspect a spinal injury always call an ambulance. If someone has an accident, a fall or car crash, for example, don't try to move them if you suspect he or she has a spinal injury.

SPLINTERS

Any type of reasonably small foreign body or material trapped under the skin can be called a splinter.

Signs and Symptoms

Pain and tenderness. A splinter may or may not be visible to the naked eye.

First Aid

If a splinter can be easily removed with a clean needle or tweezers, then it should be. But if it's embedded deeper under the skin and would mean you had to dig around to get it out, then a nurse or doctor should deal with it. However, if a splinter is left, in most cases nature will work its wonders. There will be a softening of the tissue around the splinter and secretion of liquid in reaction to the foreign body. If there are germs on the splinter, pus will be produced. (Pus is the usually yellow liquid that forms as the body's defence cells and chemical antibodies arrive at the wound site and do battle. The extra blood supply to this part causes some liquid to escape into and out of the wound, carrying with it dead, dying and living germs and tissue fluids.) In both cases, the redness and activity that follows works the splinter towards the surface of the skin so that it will eventually be easy to remove or will simply come out on its own.

STAB WOUNDS

Stab wounds, or wounds from other sharp objects such as a pair of scissors or knitting needle, for instance, can cause great damage because not only are the protective layers of skin damaged, there is a very real danger that the body's organs may be injured, too. That's why any type of stab wound or deep puncture wound (see page 178) needs prompt medical attention.

❗ Signs and Symptoms

A deep cut with profuse bleeding.

➕ First Aid

Call for medical help and staunch the flow of blood by applying pressure around the wound with a clean cloth while you're waiting for help to arrive or while accompanying the casualty to hospital. Treat for shock (see page 180).

STIES IN THE EYE

A stye is an infection at the base of an eyelash, rather like a boil.

❗ Signs and Symptoms

You may first notice some pain or feel a slight swelling at the edge of the eyelid. As the stye develops or bursts you may notice a discharge of pus.

➕ First Aid

Most styes will heal on their own if left alone. Usually they burst, seep pus or just dry up of their own accord in the course of a week.

If the stye bursts, carefully clean the eye area using a fresh piece of cotton wool moistened in cooled, previously boiled water, wiping the closed eyelid. Always wash your hands if you have touched the stye to prevent spreading any infection. Keep to your own face flannels and towels too. If the stye does not heal within seven days or so, seek your doctor's advice. The same advice applies if the stye or your eye itself becomes red and painful.

If sties become frequent do see your doctor as you may need an antibiotic ointment for just inside your nose, which could be the source of the bacteria.

STITCH

I'm sure most people will have had a stitch at some time in their lives – that sharp kind of pain felt in the abdomen. It is due to cramp in the diaphragm and tends to affect children and young people more than adults.

🛈 Signs and Symptoms

Sharp pain often seeming to come from the muscles of the abdominal wall.

➕ First Aid

First aid for a stitch, like many other problems involving muscles, is to sit down and rest until the pain subsides – which it will fairly quickly.

STOMACH ULCERS

There are two terms used when discussing ulcer problems – duodenal and gastric. The term 'peptic ulcer' is the general name for the common type of ulcer. A gastric ulcer is a peptic ulcer in the stomach and a duodenal ulcer is a peptic ulcer in the duodenum.

The stomach and duodenum separately secrete powerful juices containing hydrochloric acid and the enzyme pepsin to digest the food – especially the protein – that we eat. Normally the lining membrane of the digestive system is protected from these juices by a gel-like coating of mucus and natural antacid secretions produced by the lining cells. Sometimes, however, probably due to a complex interaction of hereditary, emotional and environmental factors, the balance is upset, the protective barrier penetrated and part of the lining (which is itself protein) is 'digested' or eroded – resulting in an ulcer.

Recently it has come to light that a germ – the Helicobacter Pylori – may be in greater part responsible. So peptic ulcers can now be cured by a relatively short course of antibiotic treatment in a medicine cocktail that also includes the acid stoppers – called the H2 antagonists – and a varying combination of differ-

Did you know?
At least one in ten people will suffer from peptic ulcers in their lifetime especially if someone in their family has done so. We tend to think they only affect high-powered businessmen in stressful jobs but research shows that they actually occur more often in the less well-off. Although duodenal ulcers are about four times more common in men, gastric ulcers affect men and women almost equally and tend to occur in later life.

ent antibiotics and perhaps bismuth. This type of treatment not only cures most peptic ulcer sufferers, but up to nineteen out of twenty of them will still remain cured after one year. Sometimes peptic ulcers, or at least gastritis – an inflammation of the stomach lining – can be caused as a consequence of other drug treatments such as the non-steroidal anti-inflammatory drugs used to treat arthritis.

❗ Signs and Symptoms

How will you know if you have an ulcer? A burning or gnawing pain felt in the middle, just below the ribs, is the main symptom. Usually the pain occurs in bouts lasting a few days or weeks, then disappears to recur several months later, the frequency of attacks tending to increase. There may also be nausea or vomiting, loss of appetite and a feeling of fullness.

Typically, the pain of a duodenal ulcer occurs between meals and is relieved by eating. Often it will wake the sufferer at night, whereas pain from a gastric ulcer rarely does so and is usually felt during, or soon after, a meal. Occasionally an ulcer will erode a blood vessel and cause bleeding, or, more rarely still, perforate the wall of the stomach or duodenum and an operation will then be vital.

➕ First Aid

Do consult a doctor if you have recurrent symptoms such as those described. Investigations, such as a barium meal or an endoscopy – a look down inside through a special flexible tube, inserted through the mouth – may be needed to make a definite diagnosis.

STRAINS, SPRAINS AND PULLED MUSCLES

A strain is a slight tearing of a muscle or the tendon attaching it to a bone, usually caused by overstretching it, whereas a sprain is a tear in a joint capsule or its supportive ligaments, due to twisting or forcing the joint beyond its normal range of movement.

However, these terms are used quite loosely even by doctors when they know they are dealing with a type of injury that is going to get better on its own whether it's treated or not – as most sprains or strains do, given time.

Other soft tissue problems include capsulitis (inflammation of a joint lining due to a twisting or jarring injury), bursitis (inflammation of the fluid-filled bursae which act as cushions at points of wear and tear) and epicondylitis (inflammation where muscle tendons join the bony points of the elbow). If pain and tenderness are on the outer point, epicondylitis is commonly known as tennis elbow (see page 209), if on the inner side, golfer's elbow, but any activity that overuses these tendons can cause the same symptoms – painting a ceiling or hammering, for example. The characteristic overuse of one particular movement of the arm, in particular, inflames the tendons that make the movement and known as tendonitis.

🛈 Signs and Symptoms

When a strain or sprain first occurs, chemicals are released into the damaged tissues – they include prostaglandins, which sensitise nerve endings – and cause pain, inflammation and swelling.

➕ First Aid

Medicines known as NSAIDs – non-steroidal anti-inflammatory drugs – such as aspirin and ibuprofen, act to prevent or cut down the release of prostaglandins and the sooner they can be given after an injury the better.

Ibuprofen is also available as a cream or gel and studies show that it relieves pain and other symptoms when rubbed directly into the injured area, without the risk of side-effects that tablets may cause – nausea, for example.

First aid measures in the initial forty-eight hours after injury can be very helpful and speed recovery. An ice pack will reduce bruising and swelling and will also relieve pain. Wrap the ice in a wet cloth or flannel to protect the skin from iceburn and frostbite and apply the pack to the injured part for ten minutes every few hours. Contrary to popular belief, a hot bath will make matters worse, because it speeds up the flow of blood and increases swelling.

Rest the injured part as much as possible and raise it to reduce swelling (support an injured arm in a sling, for example). A compression bandage such as tubigrip, worn continuously for at least two days, will help, too, but watch for numbness, tingling or the skin colour changing to white or blue – signs that the bandage is too tight.

Prevention

Ideally, try to prevent injury occurring in the first place. Exercise, though undoubtedly good for you, should not be overdone. If you are unaccustomed to it, expert tuition is often advisable and do take things gradually to begin with. Warming up before taking any form of strenuous exercise, and warming down afterwards, is always advisable.

STROKES

Put simply a stroke is the clotting or bursting of a blood vessel in the brain which can cause paralysis. A stroke itself is a clinical description of a collection of symptoms and danger signs as a result of an underlying disease or problem. That's why there is an extremely wide range of symptoms from the mild to the very serious. What this means is that part of the brain is suddenly damaged by a blood clot or haemorrhage, depriving it of its vital blood supply. In Britain it's thought that around 100,000 people suffer strokes for the first time each year. A quarter of these strokes occur in people who are under sixty-five. Strokes vary in their intensity and effects. They are likely to cause a weakness, or even paralysis of the arm and leg on either side of the body, the face can become twisted, and sometimes there will be loss of balance, vision disturbances, speech difficulties and incontinence. At the worst end of the scale a stroke can cause loss of consciousness or confusion.

❗ Signs and Symptoms

Warning signs that a person is having a stroke are feeling very faint and giddy, accompanied by blurred vision and confusion. It can be difficult for the sufferer to speak, they may have a headache (usually severe) and they may complain of tingling in a leg or a changed sensation – pins and needles, for instance. Usually the symptoms will be contained to one side of the body since the Cerebro Vascular Accident – as the thrombosis or haemorrhage into the brain is called – occurs on one side of the brain. (Each side of the brain serves the opposite side of the body.)

➕ First Aid

You must call emergency medical help and get the person into the recovery position (see page 18). If the casualty falls unconscious you'll need to spring into action quickly with resuscitation procedures (see page 211).

🏃 Prevention

How can you prevent the risk of a stroke? If you suffer from coronary heart disease or have had heart failure, you are more likely to suffer from a stroke than someone who hasn't. High blood pressure, in part caused by smoking, heavy drinking, lack of exercise, high cholesterol levels, being overweight, high blood sugar, are all factors which put you more at risk. Most of these factors are all linked to a fatty build up known as atheroma. A build up of fat inside the arteries leads to a narrowing of the blood vessels – if this happens to the blood vessels to the heart it can lead to a heart attack and to those to the brain a stroke.

Blood pressure can be reduced by medication but most

Opportunistic testing

Nowadays, most doctors will take the opportunity to test for the otherwise unnoticeable risk factors whenever the opportunity arises. It's called opportunistic testing, which means that when someone of mature years comes to the surgery for whatever reason, the opportunity is taken to check their blood pressure and perhaps even do a blood test. Many doctors will now routinely test for known risk factors and may send out letters requesting that their patients, of a certain age and gender, come forward for these routine screening tests. This is to try to pre-empt problems before they have caused any symptoms and hopefully prevent conditions caused by high blood pressure or treat others while they are still curable.

doctors also fully appreciate the need to treat blood pressure by natural means whenever possible. These include advising the patient to lose weight, give up smoking, cut down on salt and on fatty foods and avoid excessive alcohol (which are all things that put you at risk of a stroke anyway), and to try to take some form of exercise. In this country, we, on average, eat far too much salt. This is because our tastebuds are used to it. While it's difficult to prove it is actually causing harm – though I believe it is – there is proof that for someone whose blood pressure is already too high, excess salt will make it even higher. Consequently, the chance of a stroke becomes greater.

Just by eating a balanced diet, you will take in more than enough salt for health. Pre-cooked and processed foods nearly always have extra salt added, so avoiding those is a help, as is not adding salt to cooking or at the table. This will cut the average salt intake by a quarter.

✸ After a stroke

Although basic intelligence is usually unaltered, speech, movement, memory and reading or writing abilities may all be affected for a time. However, as the clot dissolves, or the haemorrhage is drained – when possible – or gradually absorbed,

> *Cigarettes and strokes*
> According to the Stroke Association, people realise that they are at risk of developing lung cancer when they smoke cigarettes, but fail to realise that for people who smoke twenty cigarettes a day the chances of having a stroke are about three times greater than for those who do not smoke.

much of the previous function often returns. Patient persistence will be needed to practise repetitively special exercises to relearn lost skills. Plenty of encouragement, praise and calm reassurance from carers will help considerably.

Improvement is most noticeable in the first few months but can continue long after that, much depending on the individual's determination to succeed. It is often difficult but important for the carer to strike the right balance between helping with daily tasks such as dressing and undressing and encouraging the person to do things for him or herself – however slowly at first – and so regain their independence.

Visits from friends, regular outings and encouragement to resume previous interests and activities, as much as possible, all help prevent depressing isolation and feelings of uselessness.

It is thought that half of strokes could, and therefore should, be prevented and that most of those that do occur could be made less disabling with specialist treatment and rehabilitation methods begun almost at once. For example, frequent checks to see that the affected limbs, hands and feet are correctly positioned are important from the very beginning so that the muscles do not contract and cause a lasting deformity.

✳ Transient Ischaemia Attack

When someone has what appears to be a stroke but the symptoms clear up in less than an hour or so, a Transient Ischaemia Attack will often be diagnosed. The doctor may recommend that the patient takes a small dose of aspirin every day from then on – usually from a quarter to a whole tablet. This stops the blood's small platelet cells sticking together so easily and can help to prevent a subsequent thrombosis, which may well lead to a clot forming and possibly cause a proper stroke.

STUPOR

There are many causes of stupor. Too much alcohol, the aftermath of an epileptic convulsion, a recent head injury, a major organ failure such as liver failure, an overdose of drugs, or the onset of a diabetic coma may all need to be considered.

❗ Signs and Symptoms

When a person doesn't answer questions very easily, or does not seem to make sense when they try to speak, he or she may be in a state of stupor.

➕ First Aid

Seek medical help without delay unless the cause is known and the treatment obvious – like sobering up a drunken raver. If in doubt still seek medical help. Drink and drugs in overdose are well-known killers.

SUFFOCATION

Suffocation occurs when air is prevented from entering a person's airways. Asphyxiation occurs when there isn't enough oxygen in the inhaled air to support life.

❗ Signs and Symptoms

An obstruction to the airways from a carrier bag over the head, for example, can cause death by suffocation, whereas someone who attempts or achieves suicide by piping a car's exhaust fumes into the car dies from asphyxiation. Their inspired air contains too much carbon monoxide and not enough oxygen.

➕ First Aid

Your first step is to remove what is obstructing the air supply. If a carrier bag is causing the obstruction, for example, just quickly rip it open rather than try to pull it off over the casualty's head. If the person has stopped breathing follow resuscitation procedures (see Mouth-to-Mouth Resuscitation, page 16). Then place the casualty in the recovery position while awaiting medical help.

> **BE CAREFUL!**
> All types of carrier bags should be kept away from babies and young children.

SUICIDE ATTEMPTS

According to the Royal College of Psychiatrists around 5000 people commit suicide every year in the UK – many due to depression, and one in twenty adults suffers from depression at any one time.

Sometimes the desire to end it all becomes so strong in a person that they begin to plan ways of killing themselves. This is a strong indication that they need help urgently. There is no easy way to determine who is most likely to do it – even experienced psychiatrists can get it wrong. The only safe way to deal with the problem if you have suspicions that someone may commit suicide is to discuss it with their doctor. If there is reason to believe that the person has a definite mental illness and that they are at risk, they can legally be taken to a hospital for treatment and their own protection, whether they agree or not.

✳ DRUG OVERDOSE

Speed is essential when dealing with any type of drug overdose. The doses of prescribed medications are based on the lowest amounts of the drug that will have a satisfactory effect, taking into account the natural differences between people. It may surprise readers to know, that, for some medicines, the rate and speed at which the drug can be absorbed and metabolised (or used) in the body can vary by as much as eight times from person to person.

So in the case of someone who's a fast absorber but a slow metaboliser, for example, he or she may be receiving more than the dose that's necessary for the medicine to be effective.

However, they're still within safe limits if they've taken no more than the recommended dose.

And of course, it's difficult to know whether a casualty is the type of person who absorbs medicines faster than usual or who breaks them down more slowly than usual.

❗ Signs and Symptoms

Warnings signs of a drug overdose are unconsciousness, nausea and vomiting, confusion or deliriousness and sleepiness.

➕ First Aid

If you think someone has taken an overdose of painkillers or sleeping tablets, for example, always seek medical help. Put the casualty in the recovery position (see page 18) while waiting for help if they are drowsy.

Overdosage of a particular drug will occasionally have a particular antidote. That's why it's important to keep any drugs or other ingested material found nearby so that it can be identified. There is a poison reference centre where doctors can phone to seek help in identifying unusual drugs or tablets found at the scene and in discovering the specific antidote if there is one. The general approach will often be to 'wash the stomach out'. This is done by a trained person, usually a doctor or a nurse, either passing a solution down into the stomach and sucking it out again – hopefully containing enough of the ingested medicine to remove most if not all of the danger – or, more often, by giving a solution of charcoal to drink.

✳ STRANGULATION

If someone has tried to strangle or hang themselves their air supply will have been obstructed because of pressure on the neck.

❗ Signs and Symptoms

The skin will probably have become blue, breathing difficult and the veins on the face and neck will be standing out.

✚ First Aid

Remove whatever is obstructing the breathing by quickly cutting the rope or scarf they have used as a means to commit suicide. Once you have freed them the now open airway will be all that's usually needed if the person has been reached in time.

You may have to follow resuscitation procedures (see Mouth-to-Mouth Resuscitation, page 16). If they are breathing but are not conscious you'll need to put the victim in the recovery position (see page 18) while waiting for medical help to arrive.

❋ CARBON MONOXIDE INHALATION

❗ Signs and Symptoms

The casualty's breathing is likely to be quick, the skin will look blue and they may be unconscious.

✚ First Aid

If you find someone trying to commit suicide by, say, letting their car engine fumes fill the garage, you need to get yourself and the casualty out into the fresh air as quickly as possible. If they aren't breathing give mouth-to-mouth resuscitation (page 16). If unconscious, place in the recovery position (see page 18) and call for medical help.

❋ SLASHED WRISTS

✚ First Aid

Press the bleeding points with a clean cloth to quench the bleeding. Call for medical help immediately. If they are unconscious or shocked, see pages 211 and 180.

SUNBURN

If you suffer from sunburn, the painful effects don't normally last for more than a few days, followed by itching as the skin heals.

❗ Signs and Symptoms

Overexposure to the ultra-violet rays of the sun makes the skin red, hot and sore. Higher doses lead to inflammation and swelling; even greater exposure leads to burning, blistering and peeling as the epidermis – the outer layer of skin – disintegrates.

➕ First Aid

Lotions containing calamine or aloe vera with perhaps menthol, phenol or camphor have a cooling effect on the skin. If you don't have any lotions, cool the skin by applying a sponge moistened with cold water.

Blisters should not be burst and you should drink plenty of water just in case you have become dehydrated. If the skin is burnt or peeling, stay out of the sun until it has healed completely. If symptoms are severe, always consult a doctor.

BE CAREFUL!

Make sure you or your children don't pick at sunburned areas of skin. Sunburn is no different from any other burn. The skin will flake or fall off as soon as the underlayer is ready, and if you pick it off before, you will be pulling away the tender underskin that is forming, causing it to bleed It is then also more likely to heal leaving patchy areas of discoloration.

🪧 Prevention

With the proven risk of skin cancer caused by the sun's harmful rays, and the obvious ageing effects of the sun on the skin, it is more sensible to avoid getting sunburnt in the first place. The most important time to stay out of the direct sun is around midday when it's at its strongest. And always wear a hat in the sun.

It is also wise to use a medium to high-factor sunscreen – depending on your skin's sensitivity – when out and about in the sun. Apply it at least every two to three hours and after swimming. For those with very sensitive skin, a total sunscreen is strongly advised, as is covering up, because even under a sunshade you can still get burnt by the rays that bounce off the things surrounding you, such as sand, buildings and water.

Don't forget that babies and young children are particularly vulnerable to the sun's harmful rays, so always use a sun protection cream designed for their delicate skins (ask your pharmacist for advice). Babies under six months old should be kept out of the sun anyway, not just because of the risk of sunburn, but because heat stroke can be even more dangerous (see page 142).

SWALLOWING DIFFICULTIES

Sometimes elderly members of the family may find difficulty in swallowing solid food. There is quite a common condition called globus hystericus whereby, especially during times of emotion and stress, the throat muscles go into spasm. This causes a feeling of fullness in the throat and makes swallowing seem difficult.

There are several other conditions which can cause similar symptoms – a pharyngeal pouch, for example. In this case, as the small muscles which encircle the throat become lax with age, the force of swallowing pushes the lining membrane of the throat outwards to form a pouch through its muscular wall – a bit like a 'blow-out' in the inner tube of a bicycle tyre. Food may then collect in the pouch from time to time, cause pressure on the throat and interfere with swallowing. It is usually possible – by eating softer foods, for example – to overcome the problem and avoid the need for an operation.

Also, a hiatus hernia (see page 143) – which may have only caused mild symptoms – can, over the years, lead to a narrowing in the lower end of the oesophagus (gullet) as scar tissue develops. This is due to the acid gastric juices seeping upwards and producing chronic irritation. A disease of the oesophagus, called achalsia (or cardiospasm), is yet another possible cause of swallowing difficulties and is also affected by emotional upsets.

✚ First Aid

It is always essential to consult a doctor about symptoms like this.

SWALLOWING POISONS

The main thing when poison has been swallowed is to seek medical advice urgently even if – as may be the case with paracetamol poisoning, for instance – there are no apparent adverse effects at first.

If the victim is unconscious place them in the recovery position (see page 18) until help arrives because he or she could vomit at any time.

❗ Signs and Symptoms

Warning signs that someone might have swallowed a harmful substance include loss of consciousness, confusion, stomach pains, skin burns and vomiting. There may also be a staining of the skin around the mouth.

✚ First Aid

✳ Tablets and medicines

If you're not sure whether a child, for example, has swallowed something, spend a minute or two quickly searching for any missing pills or containers nearby. Don't forget to look under tables or chairs in case the container or pills have rolled away. Having said that, don't spend too long searching.

It's best to take your child or older casualty to your doctor or hospital Accident and Emergency unit – whichever is the quickest. If possible, always take a sample or the container of whatever liquid or medicines you think may have been swallowed.

✲ Household and garden chemicals, bleach, turps, white spirit, fertilisers, etc

Calmly give the child or older casualty a glass of milk to drink. Liquid like this helps to dilute the poison. If you don't have any milk, water will do. Even eating some ice cream can help.

Never use salt and water to make the child sick. If the swallowed substance was corrosive vomiting could cause further harm. If vomiting occurs naturally, keep a sample to show to the doctor.

Once that's done, you'll need to get the casualty to hospital as soon as you can, taking with you whatever substance you suspect might have been swallowed. An antidote will be given or the stomach will be washed out, or other types of treatment will be used, depending on the circumstances.

Did you know?

You would probably be amazed if you added up the total number of poisonous substances in your home. Commonly used solutions like bleach, paint stripper and thinner, paraffin, methylated spirit, white spirit, lighter fuel, oven cleaner, lavatory cleaner and window cleaning fluid can be lethal if swallowed by a young child. Alcohol, of course, is potentially a poison and, perhaps surprisingly, Mummy's favourite perfume can contain enough alcohol to be harmful if a toddler drinks it. Other dangerous substances found in many homes include deodorants, insecticides, weedkiller, fertiliser, antifreeze, hair lacquer, caustic soda, glue, paints and varnish. And that's without mentioning medicines.

Every year some 40,000 people – mainly children – are taken to hospital with accidental poisoning. One survey found that gardening and motoring chemicals were the most dangerous, followed by cleaning and DIY chemicals. The most dangerous storage areas were sheds, greenhouses and utility rooms, followed by garages and kitchens and, lastly, bathrooms.

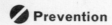
Prevention

Poisoning in adults is more often than not deliberate, rather than accidental as it is with children. All parents, for instance, have heard the message, time and time again, that pills, potions and medicines should be out of sight of inquisitive children. But no matter how many times it's said, it really is essential to keep harmful substances out of reach, under lock and key and whenever possible in childproof containers. Also, don't hoard medicines – return them to your pharmacist for disposal. Kitchen cleaners, loo cleaners and the like should be kept in a cupboard with a childproof catch. Don't leave alcohol around either. It too could prove tempting for youngsters who won't realise the consequences of drinking it. Children under the age of two are at the greatest risk of swallowing a harmful substance.

All too often children are far too young to understand the implications of their curiosity. Even something as innocuous as vitamin tablets can be harmful to a child. Multivitamin tablets, for example, can include iron and this can be dangerous for any youngster. The child will need professional medical help, and in all likelihood have his or her stomach pumped out.

A good piece of advice would be not to take tablets or medicine in front of a young child. They may want to copy you doing that, just as they may want to copy you in lots of other less harmful ways. Explain to older children the effects that medicines and poisonous chemicals can have – just forbidding them to touch may only act as a challenge!

Another good piece of advice is that it's important to always keep household chemicals in their original containers. White spirit, for instance, if transferred to a lemonade bottle can look like a tempting drink to a small child. If labels have come off a container and you are unsure what is inside, it's best to throw it away.

SWALLOWING FOREIGN OBJECTS

Children have been known to swallow coins, marbles and small toys or parts of toys. Such substances aren't poisonous and won't obstruct breathing, but you'll need to consult the doctor who may possibly want an X-ray to find out where the object is and to determine whether it could cause any damage internally. In most cases you'll just have to let the digestive system take its course and the foreign object will be passed in a day or two.

SWOLLEN ANKLES

It's relatively common for women, in particular, to suffer from swollen ankles. However, if you're fit in every other way, it's unlikely that there's a serious problem, such as heart, kidney or blood disease.

❗ Signs and Symptoms

Swelling around the ankles, caused by the tissues becoming 'bogged' with fluid which accumulates when a person has to stand still for long periods, as is often the case in shop work.

➕ First Aid

If your ankles are swollen take off your shoes and rest with your legs elevated above your waist.

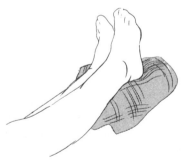

Prevention

Walking or cycling to work will activate your muscles and so help reduce swelling. When you have a break, sit with your legs raised to just above waist level.

Try graduated support stockings (on NHS prescription) or tights (available from pharmacies), which help to keep swelling to a minimum, and move about as much as possible while at work. If you're overweight, aim to lose excess pounds to relieve the pressure on your ankles. Swollen ankles can also be a side-effect of your medication so check with your pharmacist.

Finally, reduce the salt intake in your diet. Even if you don't add salt to dishes, you could still be consuming it in processed foods so check labels before buying.

TEETHING

Babies cut their first teeth, on average, at about the age of six months and complete their set of twenty baby or milk teeth when they're around two to three years old. The first don't usually give any trouble, but when the back teeth come through they can cause pain.

! Signs and Symptoms

Teething trouble is pretty easy to spot – if your baby is grisly or upset, dribbling more than usual, has red cheeks or is gnawing everything in reach, then it's likely that teething is the cause. But if you have any doubts at all, it's best to get medical advice so as not to blame teething and overlook any real illness.

+ First Aid

Special teething gels are available to relieve the baby's discomfort and you can apply it using a small pad of cotton wool or a clean finger. Rub the baby's gums gently. If your child is in great discomfort you can also use paracetamol infant suspensions to relieve the pain.

Did you know?
Nowadays it's unfashionable to consider that teething is the cause of any symptoms. Who wants to be fashionable!

TENNIS ELBOW

Tennis elbow is thought to be due to an inflammation of the tendon attached to the muscles which pull the hand backwards and twist it outwards. It is similar to other soft tissue injuries in the body caused either by regular overuse or by sudden excessive use of the tendon.

Other vulnerable places are the inside of the elbow (golfer's elbow) and the top of the shoulder, where the tendon raising the arm sideways acts as a pulley. The problem can also occur where the tendon attached to the lower end of the knee cap becomes inflamed (patella tendinitis); or on the bottom of the foot, when the tough sheet of fibres under the skin is involved; or at the back of the ankle where the Achilles tendon is situated. The former is usually known as a spur heel.

Some specialists think these inflamed tendons may be due not just to overuse, but to a restriction in blood supply to the affected tendon, making it weak and more easily strained.

While the condition can occur in someone who plays tennis or does any other repetitive movement for the first time in a long while, it can also happen to a very fit and highly trained athlete, suggesting that there's something more than strain involved.

🛑 Signs and Symptoms

Inflammation and pain around the elbow.

➕ First Aid

If you think you have tennis elbow, rest is the body's way to heal inflamed tissues – and pain is the signal telling you to rest! It's almost always inadvisable to ignore pain, unless it's on the advice of a trained professional. Passive exercise, usually using the good arm to move the affected arm gently, will prevent other muscles and the elbow joint from stiffening.

Fortunately, for the majority of people, most attacks of tennis elbow will go away on their own, given time. It may be useful in some cases to seek professional help. Skilled massage and treatments such as ultrasound and pulsed high-frequency electro-magnetic energy (PEME) should bring deep relief.

Good advice on rest and exercise is invaluable.

Sometimes, if the exact spot can be discovered where the inflammation is greatest, an injection of a powerful anti-inflammatory, such as hydro-cortisone, may bring considerable if not total relief very quickly.

If the condition becomes chronically persistent, then surgeons may decide to operate to remove the attachment of the inflamed tendon and re-attach it to the bone. This is not often necessary, but can be useful in a few cases. However it is only used as a last resort and in the most persistent cases.

TRAVEL SICKNESS

See Holiday First Aid, page 226.

TWISTING AN ANKLE

Twists and sprains in an ankle are easily done.

❗ Signs and Symptoms

Pain around the ankle area, particularly on movement.

✚ First Aid

The best medicine for most sprains and strains is rest. If you have hurt your ankle, you should rest it with your foot up, preferably raised above your waist. (See also Strains, Sprains and Pulled Muscles, page 193.)

TWISTED TESTICLE

Many parents may not realise that one medical emergency for a boy child is the twisting – or torsion – of a testicle out of its normal position. It's an emergency because torsion will cut off the testicle's blood supply and you must act immediately to prevent permanent damage and even loss of the testicle.

❗ Signs and Symptoms

This can happen without any obvious cause and can be very painful indeed. Warning signs of such an emergency can be unexplained pain and swelling accompanied by redness of the testicle. There may be nausea and vomiting, as well as shock. Or the symptoms may not be very dramatic – just unaccustomed pain.

✚ First Aid

Don't give the child anything to eat or drink because of the possibility of surgery. Just keep calm and don't show just how concerned you are. You must get your child to your GP as soon as possible. He may refer you to an A&E department where a doctor will try to untwist the testicle. If it can't be untwisted by gentle manipulation surgery will be required.

UNCONSCIOUSNESS

Unconsciousness means that though the casualty is breathing and has a heartbeat, he or she still cannot be roused.

✚ First Aid

If a person is unconscious:

1 Always put them in the recovery position (see page 18).
2 Once in the recovery position it's then safer for you to get medical help, although it is advisable not to leave any unconscious casualty alone because he or she may stop breathing or choke.
3 If they stop breathing you must give mouth-to-mouth resuscitation (see page 16).
4 If the heart stops beating you will need to give heart massage (see page 13) as well.

VOMITING

Vomiting and nausea are very common symptoms. Causes include a stomach germ, early pregnancy, travel sickness, eating and drinking too much, gastric disorders and a reaction to cancer therapy. Careful enquiry needs to be made to ascertain why a person is suffering in this way and a likely diagnosis made before appropriate treatment and advice can be given.

Signs and Symptoms

The involuntary emptying of the stomach.

First Aid

For 'straightforward' vomiting that seems to be the result of a tummy bug or travel sickness, or of eating something that hasn't agreed with them (or of perhaps eating too much of something in the case of a child), then offer sips of water or one of the rehydrating mixtures supplied by the pharmacy. Advise the sufferer to rest for a while until he or she feels better.

BE CAREFUL!

Do seek your doctor's advice if there is also abdominal pain, headache, severe diarrhoea, or blood in the vomit, or if the vomiting continues for what seems to be an excessive length of time, or if the vomit contains food that was eaten more than four hours previously.

WASP STINGS

All insects are either biters or stingers. When a bee stings, it generally leaves its sting in place and flies off without it. A wasp sticks its stinging tail into its victim and injects its irritant substance.

Many irritant substances – like the venom in a wasp or hornet's sting – can stimulate the body into a more severe reaction the next time it is confronted with a similar substance. Bees or wasps can cause the sufferer to react in this way, although wasps seem to be the main culprit, as people are stung more often by them than they are by bees.

Signs and Symptoms

Pain, redness or swelling.

First Aid

As a wasp does not leave its sting behind, you'll just need to treat a sting with an application of a teaspoonful of vinegar in half a tumbler of water. Any remaining pain can be treated with common painkillers or antihistamine tablets.

Stings around the mouth or nose can sometimes swell and interfere with breathing. In extreme cases, if there is a reaction, a person may collapse. In severe situations like these, get medical help immediately. As in bee stings (see page 42) if a child under two gets stung, seek medical advice anyway.

Prevention

If you are susceptible, you may be advised to avoid wasp-plagued places. Your doctor may also give you an injection to carry with you. If stung again, you can administer a shot yourself.

What can you do if you love eating outside during the summer, but your garden always seems to have more than its fair share of wasps, and you inevitably get stung? First, stay calm. They will only sting if they are attacked or feel threatened – which they will if you flap your hands at them! Above all, don't let yourself get so worked up about them that they spoil your summer.

WHIPLASH INJURY

A whiplash injury is a sudden jarring of the spine which occurs when the head is jerked backwards and forwards either in a collision – in a car crash, for example – or in a fall – while skiing, for instance.

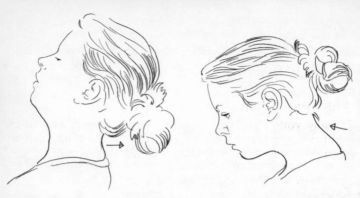

ⓘ Signs and Symptoms

The jarring bruises and inflames the nerves leading from the upper part of the spinal cord and this causes the pain around the neck and other symptoms. The pain will often take hours or a day or so before it starts.

➕ First Aid

In the meantime rest and consult your doctor. He may consider prescribing muscle relaxants to keep at least some of the oncoming muscle spasm at bay.

Wearing a neck collar restricts movement of the head and neck and allows the inflammation to subside more quickly. I'm afraid it may take several months to do so and some arthritis may develop in that part of the neck in later years. Anti-inflammatory medicines, such as aspirin or ibuprofen, should help.

The risk of long-term problems is reduced if physiotherapy is begun early on.

⊘ Prevention

The chances of having a whiplash injury are greatly reduced if you always use headrests, as well as the compulsory fastening of seatbelts, in your car.

WHOOPING COUGH

Incidents of whooping cough are now becoming less common as more and more children are immunised (see page 149).

⚠ Signs and Symptoms

Initially your child may seem to be starting a cold (high temperature, sneezing, runny nose) followed by uncontrollable coughing with a noisy intake of breath and vomiting.

➕ First Aid

Contact your GP as soon as possible. Antibiotics can reduce the severity of symptoms if prescribed early. If a child turns blueish or has trouble breathing, get them to hospital at once.

WRIST, SPRAINED

Sprains of the wrist are soft tissue injuries. See also page 193.

⚠ Signs and Symptoms

Pain and inflammation around the wrist.

➕ First Aid

It may help to rest your wrist if you bandage it with a crepe bandage, or a lighter type called a retention bandage.

Did you know?
Don't remove the crepe bandage at night. When you are asleep you are unaware of the position your injured wrist could be in, even if that position might otherwise cause you pain. The idea of a crepe bandage is to act as an additional support to those tissues that normally support the wrist, allowing them to heal more quickly. Don't make it too tight though.

215

PART

3

HOLIDAY FIRST AID

Each summer I seem to be asked what you need to take with you on holiday 'just in case'. Having a good first aid kit with you can save a lot of time, trouble and expense. It's best to ask your pharmacist's advice on suitable remedies for very young children but for older children and adults the kit could include:

* soluble aspirin and/or paracetamol
* insect repellent
* antihistamine tablets for preventing travel sickness, and treating mild sunburn and stings
* sun protection creams of various factor strengths
* calamine lotion for soothing sunburn or insect bites
* waterproof sticking plasters
* water-purifying tablets
* indigestion and constipation remedies
* a good supply of any medicine you may be taking
* mineral and glucose replacement treatments for simple diarrhoea or vomiting. Some pharmacists supply bowel quieteners such as Arret.

ADVERSE EFFECTS OF THE SUN

A bright sunny day makes most people feel better and the warmth of the sun is comforting. But both of these are emotional benefits and, because they make us feel good, we automatically assume that the sun's ultraviolet A (UVA) rays are naturally good for us. The truth is, they rarely are. This is none more relevant than when we are on holiday and have the opportunity to spend more time in the sun. Always increase your exposure to the sun gradually. See also Sunburn, page 202.

Signs and Symptoms

Sore, hot, red skin. Headaches.

➕ First Aid

If you have a little too much sun, make sure you drink plenty of water to prevent dehydration and apply a soothing aftersun cream or calamine lotion to help take the heat out of sore skin. See also Heat Illnesses, page 142.

DOG BITES

If you are bitten by a dog while on holiday abroad you need to seek medical advice and possibly have an anti-rabies injection. Otherwise follow the general measures outlined under Dog Bites, see page 100.

EARACHE WHEN FLYING

One problem you might encounter when you're travelling to your holiday destination, if you are going by plane, is earache caused by pressure changes.

The changes in air pressure following a take-off and during descent mean air contained in the body can increase in volume by almost a third. The chances are that pain is due to congestion in the small Eustachian tubes in your ears. It would seem that although they will allow air in the middle ear to escape and the pressure therefore to equalize when you ascend to the specially pressurised height of 6000 feet with the aircraft, the pressure is not able to equalise in reverse.

❗ Signs and Symptoms

Pain in the ears.

➕ First Aid

The best way of relieving the problem is by holding your nose to cut off the air supply, and blowing out through your nose at the same time until you feel air going through the passage that connects ears and throat. Swallowing, yawning or sucking a sweet can have the same effect.

220

HOLIDAY TUMMY

Most attacks of diarrhoea are caused by gastro-intestinal infections – you can think of them as the body's way of getting rid of harmful substances. If more than one member of your family suffers at the same time, it is likely the diarrhoea was caused by something you've all eaten. If you are on holiday you may be exposed to standards of hygiene that do not match up to what you are used to, resulting in what we know as 'holiday tummy' or 'gyppy tummy'. If your diarrhoea is accompanied by vomiting, food poisoning is also a likely cause. See also Diarrhoea, page 97.

⚠ Signs and Symptoms

Diarrhoea involves several loose or liquid bowel movements. It is also often accompanied by cramping pain in the lower abdomen. It can make you feel quite exhausted and if you are on holiday can ruin your fun.

✚ First Aid

Whatever the cause, most attacks of diarrhoea usually clear up quickly and without medical attention – which is good news for holiday makers. The best way to treat yourself is not eating for twenty-four hours and drinking plenty of watery drinks (no

> *Be careful! Babies at risk*
> In normally healthy adults, diarrhoea is rarely a serious condition – but children and the elderly may suffer much more. This is because they are more sensitive to the problems of dehydration and often have less body fluid to lose. Babies under six months old are at the greatest risk from dehydration – their metabolic rate is high, their kidneys don't yet retain water very efficiently and they lose a greater proportion of water compared to their weight than adults. Any baby who suffers holiday tummy should be seen by a doctor, as should an adult if symptoms persist.

Did you know?

It's not just germs you come into contact with on holiday that cause holiday tummy. The change of environment, food and emotions can all contribute to produce vomiting, stomach cramps and diarrhoea. The germs that cause gastro-intestinal upset are often the ones that are common in the community and to which the locals are immune. In the same way, visitors to this country may also experience stomach upsets – routine tests on our food and drink have revealed the presence of germs to which we've become accustomed. They don't upset us at home unless one of their more virulent 'cousins' – or pathogens – is present.

Pre-holiday inoculations protect you from many known pathogens abroad but, unfortunately, they're unable to protect you from the everyday tummy upset germs of a more humble variety.

---

milk-based products). Frequent bursts of diarrhoea can make you feel even more ill as your body becomes dehydrated. The greatest risk from diarrhoea, and from vomiting too, is that the body's essential minerals are lost at the same time, making you feel weak and eventually faint. Rehydration salts for children are now available to help prevent this.

You can also take some anti-diarrhoea medicine that you might have brought on holiday with you. If you do, you will still need to drink plenty to prevent dehydration.

If you have a problem with diarrhoea when you return from holiday, you may need to see your doctor for advice. While the symptoms of a bout of diarrhoea contracted on holiday can continue for several days – albeit becoming increasingly less severe – the fact that diarrhoea persists for more than a week suggests that a germ is responsible and of a kind that is likely to need your doctor's advice and/or treatment.

One of the most common of these germs is salmonella. With this germ and many such germs, our body's natural defences – antibodies – relieve the symptoms and destroy most of the germs, but some germs can persist for as long as a year. This means that while the germ ceases to affect its human host, it can still be passed on to others.

There are many other causes of persistent diarrhoea, often first picked up abroad. Your doctor would probably give you a specimen jar and ask you to collect a sample of your stool in order to detect the germ that could be the cause.

Prevention

To help avoid gyppy tummy and the holiday runs – or worse – be careful with the ice in those long, cool drinks. In some countries, too, you'll need to brush your teeth with bottled water and be careful about eating salads. Examples of this are when you are outside Northern Europe, North America, Australia and New Zealand, unless you're in a hotel belonging to an international chain where standards are usually guaranteed. Eat only well-cooked foods in other places. Be wary, too, of local beverages – stick to the internationally known brands if in doubt.

Avoid raw, unpeeled fruit and salads, shellfish, ice-cream – and ice if the water is suspect. Hot food, freshly cooked, is safest – the virus that causes jaundice, for instance, is killed by just one minute's boiling.

Avoid foods stored in unhygienic conditions and wash your hands frequently, especially before eating or preparing food. Having said all this, many people take holidays abroad without following any of this advice and suffer no illness! Fortunately, serious infections are now reasonably uncommon but if you go well prepared you are much more likely to have a happy and healthy holiday.

The germ responsible for most holiday tummies is often a local version of a virus.

Unfortunately, there are no effective antibiotics for viruses that invade the gut. And, even when the germs are bacterial, antibiotics are rarely effective in combating the symptoms. This is because the germs have a way of protecting themselves from the full effects of antibiotics, especially at the start of the illness when the symptoms are at their worst.

MALARIA

Malaria is a disease found in certain tropical countries. At times it can be serious but if you are travelling to a country affected by it, don't panic. In the main it can be prevented or the effects minimised by carrying out common-sense measures and taking anti-malarial tablets.

🛈 Signs and Symptoms

Fever with shivering attacks, headache and muscle pains.

➕ First Aid

Make the casualty comfortable until medical help is available.

◐ Prevention

Malaria occurs when small parasites are passed from one person to another by the bites of certain infected female mosquitoes. If you are planning a holiday, or business trip, to a malaria-prone area, do seek the advice of your doctor or recognised travel medicine service as the choice of tablets depends on the country and area you are travelling to and when you are planning to visit. If you are prescribed anti-malarial tablets (as with any other medicine) make sure you follow directions to the letter.

You'll need to take the full course – and remember that as no anti-malaria medicine is 100 per cent effective, there is a small risk that malaria can develop during or after preventive medication.

When you do travel abroad, make sure you sleep in a room that is screened against mosquitoes or that you use a mosquito net (preferably one that has been treated with an insect repellent) over the bed. Check for holes in the net, and be sure to tuck the edges under the mattress before nightfall. Use insect repellents, ointments, lotions and sprays to deter mosquitoes. In the evening, cover the arms and legs with light coloured, long-sleeved clothes and trousers. Anklets are also available which have been treated with repellent. Vaporising electric 'mats' (which give off an insect repellent aerosol), mosquito coils or tablets can be used around exposed areas of the body.

MARINE STINGS

Holidays abroad can result in stings from marine life such as corals and sea anemones or injury to the skin from standing on or inadvertently touching a sea urchin. Many of the toxins which are injected with the sting and which cause pain are heat labile – they break down with the heat and the toxin loses its effect.

Signs and Symptoms

Intense pain.

First Aid

With most such 'marine' punctures, whenever possible, put your foot in a bucket of water as hot as you can reasonably bear. And then go to a hospital or doctor.

With some of the toxins from fish spikes, especially when the fish was lying on the sand with its spines erect when you stood on it, the pain can be so intense that you'll find it well worthwhile somehow finding a bucket of hot water. If you really can't, or can't get help from a doctor or pharmacist, then the best you'll be able to do is treat the symptoms with whatever painkilling drug and antihistamine remedies you have available until you can get professional help. See also Jellyfish Stings, page 155.

PRICKLY HEAT

You may not even have suffered from prickly heat before, until you go on holiday to a hot country. Prickly heat is an extremely irritating skin rash which develops in hot weather. It occurs – more in some people than in others – when the small blood vessels under the skin widen as the temperature rises. The extra blood they then supply to the surface of the body acts as the body's radiator, allowing heat to escape. The extra blood also

225

supplies the excess liquid which the sweat glands release as sweat. As the tissues swell with blood and tissue fluids, the skin becomes congested and the pores are squeezed and then blocked. The sweat builds up under the skin and causes the red rash.

❗ Signs and Symptoms

Sufferers from prickly heat will quickly recognise the emergence of small red pimples or blisters. The tissues look red because the small blood vessels are open wide, while the engorged tissues cause discomfort and feel prickly.

➕ First Aid

There's no simple, quick first aid remedy, but if you can immerse yourself in water to keep cool, you should feel better. Covering yourself with light, white clothing will help and, obviously, keeping out of direct sunlight is a good idea, too. Calamine cream or lotions will cool the skin and antihistamine tablets can bring great relief.

TRAVEL SICKNESS

One of the worst aspects of travel sickness is the embarrassment that goes with it. This is due not only to the physical aspects of vomiting but also to the attitude of others when someone is sick in a public place. Some people are unkind to sufferers, but travel sickness deserves understanding. It can be an extremely nasty complaint, and is often unavoidable.

The cause of travel sickness has yet to be found, but it probably arises because the balance mechanism in the sufferer's inner ear is too sensitive. This is responsible for telling us where we are in relation to the ground, so constant movement produces a similar sensation to being drunk – another occasion when the balance mechanism loses its ability to tell us where we are in space. In both cases we feel nauseous and may even be sick.

The eyes also play an interesting part in all this. People whose balance mechanism does not work at all (because of nerve degeneration, for instance), can still walk and 'know where they are', provided they can see. But if such a sufferer shuts their eyes they immediately fall over and feel sick as well.

Children are particularly prone to travel sickness. It's almost as though, because their sense organs are rapidly absorbing life's information, the inner ear becomes over-sensitive. With some children, almost any movement induced by travel will make them feel ill.

Because our eyes help our inner ears judge where we are and how to keep our balance, many children feel happier in a car if they can keep their eyes on the horizon in front, rather than having their balance upset by having to look at scenery as it flashes past. The need to change focus frequently will trigger travel sickness in a great number of children.

Signs and Symptoms

Nausea and/or vomiting.

First Aid

See Vomiting, page 212.

Prevention

You can reduce the risk of travel sickness by following some self-help measures. Don't have a large meal or alcoholic drink before a journey, don't allow smoking in the car and keep windows open if possible.

If you have children who suffer, don't talk about being sick in front of them, and provide plenty of distractions – games, toys, puzzles etc. If possible, travel at night when they're more likely to fall asleep.

Providing the sufferer is not unduly sensitive to travel sickness medicines and takes them in the right dosage before the journey begins, they can be remarkably effective. The other encouraging thing is that the vast majority of people will grow out of the complaint by the time they reach their teens.

Travel sickness is not something anyone would wish on themselves – it is an overwhelming bodily reaction. So do try to be sympathetic if you are travelling with someone who is affected.

SPORTS INJURIES

The 1991 data recorded by the Leisure Accident Surveillance System revealed that out of its sample of thirteen hospitals with a twenty-four-hour Accident and Emergency department, there were more than 10,000 cases dealt with as a result of accidents on outdoor sports fields! The sport causing the most accidents was football, followed some way behind by rugby, then riding.

In the following pages I discuss some of the common first aid problems you may encounter on the sports field. See also Broken Bones (page 51) and Bruises (page 57).

CAULIFLOWER EARS

Cauliflower ears are caused by bleeding into the tissues of the external ear – the pinna – following a blow, most often while boxing or playing rugby.

Signs and Symptoms

Swelling and pain around the ear.

First Aid

At the time it occurs, if the injured ear is pressed upon with a clean cloth and then firmly bandaged against the head, can help to contain the amount of bleeding and prevent the development of a cauliflower ear. If one starts to develop, go to an Accident and Emergency department as soon as possible.

CONCUSSION

Concussion means that the brain has been bruised, albeit mildly. The brain is suspended on ligaments in a water-filled cask.

When the skull is knocked the brain bounces off the side of the knock and can hit the other side of the skull – an occurrence called coup and contrecoup. (See also page 76.)

Signs and Symptoms

Signs of concussion include a dimness of vision, a feeling of losing consciousness, a sense of feeling faint or sick, all following a head injury.

First Aid

If a person on a sports field shows signs of concussion, medical help must be called. While waiting for it to arrive, keep the casualty flat and warm with blankets, coats or whatever is available.

DEAD LEG

A blow suffered against a nerve in a limb, often the leg, can temporarily anaesthetise it. This is known as dead leg.

Signs and Symptoms

Feelings of numbness or a limb becoming temporarily immovable.

First Aid

Fortunately, the nerve will usually recover on its own and the leg will return to normal, although it may take several days or longer, depending upon the severity of the blow.

GASHES ON THE HEAD OR FACE

Gashes can sometimes occur as a result of a punch being thrown, a clash of heads, or a foul, or a stray boot. (See also Cuts and Lacerations, page 84.)

❗ Signs and Symptoms

Profuse bleeding.

➕ First Aid

If possible clean the wound by pouring fresh water over it. Then press with a clean cloth to stop further bleeding. If the gash is deep or long it may need stitches, so it should be seen by a doctor.

HAMSTRINGS

Sometimes I'm asked about knee pain following a game of squash, whether pain at the back of the knee is a ligament injury rather than damage to a muscle, and whether or not treatment will be the same. Treatment is mostly the same. Ligament, tendon or sinew all describe the hard fibrous attachment of a muscle to a bone. At the back of the knee, these tendons are known as hamstrings and they attach the powerful thigh muscles to the bones at the top of the lower leg.

❗ Signs and Symptoms

If there's a very sudden tightening of the thigh muscles and therefore the hamstrings, then either the muscle or the hamstring can overstretch and cause small tears.

BE CAREFUL!

My best advice, as with all sports, is to train properly for the level of activity you aim to achieve and, even then, to make sure you always warm up the muscles and ligaments properly before you begin exercising. You should also 'warm' them down again at the end with gentle exercise which allows the muscles to clear the chemical wastes that have built up. Just like race horses who are walked for a while after a hard run!

➕ First Aid

Treatment varies, depending on the severity of the injury and whether the sinew has been torn from its bony attachment. With minor injuries, treatment probably means applying liniment to the area and taking painkilling anti-inflammatory medicines by mouth, plus rest.

A more severe injury may need a full groin-to-ankle plaster cast to immobilise the lower limb, so the thigh and knee cannot move.

SNOW BLINDNESS

A less common sports injury is snow blindness. The dangers of the sun are known to people who enjoy summer sports but for those of us who go skiing each winter there is the risk of snow blindness. The sun's ultra-violent rays can damage your eyes as well as your skin. Sunlight will be reflected off the snow and you can be in danger of developing snow blindness if you do not wear proper goggles or sunglasses.

❗ Signs and Symptoms

Temporary blindness as the eye's cornea becomes inflamed.

➕ First Aid

Seek medical advice immediately.

TORN LIGAMENTS

Torn ligaments are common sports injuries in people who like skiing and are keen on ball games – particularly football and hockey. Sports injuries often cause damaged cartilages. They result from the jarring and twisting movements during sports such as rugby, hockey, squash, skiing and weightlifting, too. The repetitive knee movements and stresses involved in jogging, cycling and rowing, for instance, can cause problems and even jumping down on to a hard surface can damage the knee.

231

The knee and other joints in the body are at their most vulnerable when we're either crouching or straightening up – particularly if there is twisting involved. This is a common movement in football, for example, and the knee and back are more likely to be strained or sprained during this sort of game, especially if the person hasn't warmed up properly or is unfit due to lack of training.

! Signs and Symptoms

Warning signs include a painful knee that sometimes seems to 'lock' or give way.

If cartilages – the internal pads within the knee joint – are torn, they can stop the knee straightening out fully, which means that the sufferer is caught unawares when walking and the knee can let them down by locking halfway.

This locking action may not hurt some people at all, but other sufferers experience considerable pain as a result.

✚ First Aid

Take the weight off the casualty's knee and support it as comfortably as possible until medical help is available. Depending on the severity of the cartilage tear, it may heal on its own, but, if a piece is torn off, it will nearly always need removal through an arthroscope.

Likewise, a strained ligament may heal, but a tear will need surgery. Quite a lot of repair work can now be done to the knee through an arthroscope without the patient having to undergo a full operation with the knee being opened up.

WINDING

Winding can occasionally happen on the football pitch, in a rugby game or even when you've fallen on the ski slope.

! Signs and Symptoms

Pain in the upper abdomen. A feeling that the 'wind' has been knocked out of you. Any kind of blow to the upper abdomen or lower chest can cause winding. It is due to the blow to the muscles of respiration temporarily disenabling – mildly paralysing – them.

➕ First Aid

If you have been winded, just sit down wherever you can and loosen any clothing at the waist or around the chest. Then relax for a few moments. Your breathing will start again although it can be quite a frightening experience. If you're with someone to whom this happens and they lose consciousness, follow the guidance given for resuscitation on page 16.

HIV RISK IN FIRST AID

AIDS, which stands for Acquired Immune Deficiency Syndrome, is taking over from cancer as the most feared of diseases. For some this fear is based on ignorance – the mistaken belief that it can be caught, for instance, by just sitting next to or sharing crockery with an infected person or from swimming pools or lavatory seats. On the other hand, ignorance makes others too complacent: it has been apparent for some time that it is not just homosexuals and drug addicts who are at risk – anyone can catch it, man, woman or child.

Aids is due to a virus – a minute infectious germ. There are more than 300 different identified viruses and probably many more, as yet unidentified, which can cause a variety of illnesses ranging from mild – the common cold and chickenpox, for example – to severe (poliomyelitis). HIV (Human Immune Virus) is the name given to the virus responsible for AIDS.

Viruses, unlike most other germs, are not killed by antibiotics so the body must rely on its own defences to overcome them. In some cases (measles, for example) protective vaccines have been developed that will prevent the disease. When a virus, or other germ, gets into the bloodstream, special white blood cells produce antibodies to fight the invader. A specific antibody is produced in response to each different type of germ and experts are able to tell, from a blood test, which germs the body has encountered in the past from recognising the particular antibodies present in the blood.

If a blood test reveals this HIV antibody, we now know that that person may develop AIDS symptoms – usually within ten years of the initial infection.

However, the issue is confused because many with an antibody positive result have so far remained symptom-free, although are likely to be carriers of the virus and therefore potentially infectious. Another danger lies in the fact that it may take about three months after infection for antibodies to show up in a blood test – meanwhile that person is unknowingly infectious.

Preventing further spread of the virus is vital. Spread occurs when the virus from the infected blood or semen of the carrier is able to get into another's bloodstream – so an intact skin is an effective preventative barrier. The virus has been detected in other body fluids such as saliva and tears, and, although no one has yet been known to catch Aids from these, there may be, in theory, a slight risk from very passionate kissing. Once outside the body, the virus is easily destroyed by ordinary washing up and washing of clothes, for instance.

We can be assured that we will not catch AIDS from the air we breathe, or from normal social contact, so it quite unnecessary to treat an AIDS sufferer like a leper. Yet people are concerned when it comes to giving first aid to a stranger.

As far as I am concerned I would try, as I have always done, to keep to a minimum any risk of infection passing between the carer and the cared for. And by infection I mean any infection, not simply HIV. So, take all reasonable steps to avoid touching blood and body liquids and wash them off just as soon as you can. Wearing gloves, if they are to hand, can help. Ideally, every first aider should carry disposable surgical gloves – because avoiding skin to skin contact is a good practice to follow. When someone is bloodsoaked, cover them if possible with any clean cloth to hand before you handle them.

HEPATITIS B

In any case, the Hepatitis B virus – which leads to serious inflammation of the liver – is far more likely to be contracted than HIV. It is caught in identical ways to HIV, but its progress can be prevented by injections. So if you have attended a casualty, administered mouth-to-mouth resuscitation or otherwise been in contact with their 'body fluids' – blood, saliva, for example – seek medical advice.

If at all possible, avoid cutting or injuring yourself while attending an accident so that none of the casualty's blood – not even a drop – can pass through your skin and into your bloodstream. See that the sufferer's mouth is dry before giving mouth-to-mouth. Taking these precautions will ensure that the chances of catching an infection are negligible.

HELPFUL ADDRESSES

Age Concern

England
Astral House, 1268 London Road, London, SW16 4ER.
Telephone 081 679 8000.

Northern Ireland
6 Lower Crescent, Belfast, BT7 1NR.
Telephone 0232 245729.

Scotland
54A Fountainbridge, Edinburgh, EH3 9PT.
Telephone 031 228 5656.

Wales
4th Floor, 1 Cathedral Road, Cardiff, CF1 9SD.
Telephone 0222 371566.

Age Concern has a network of 1100 Age Concern groups in the United Kingdom working with volunteers to provide a variety of community services, including day centres, lunch clubs, visiting for the lonely, as well as transport and many other schemes. It has a wide range of publications for older people and those who work with them.

British Allergy Foundation
St Bartholomew's Hospital,
West Smithfield, London, EC1A 7BE.
Telephone 071 600 6127.

British Diabetic Association
10 Queen Anne Street, London, W1M OBD.
Telephone 071 323 1531.

A charity helping diabetics and supporting diabetes research.

236

British Epilepsy Association

Anstey House, 40 Hanover Square, Leeds, LS3 1BE.
Telephone 0532 439393.

A membership-based national charity which exists to help all
people with epilepsy, their families and those who care for
them. The National Information Centre and the Epilepsy
Helpline advises more than 30,000 people every year. The
helpline is 0345 089 599 (cheap rate phone line).

British Red Cross

9 Grosvenor Crescent, London, SW1X 7EJ.
Telephone 071 235 5454.

Child Accident Prevention Trust

Clerks Court, 18–20 Farringdon Lane, London, EC1R 3AU.
Telephone 071 608 3828.

The British Heart Foundation

14 Fitzhardinge Street, London W1H 4DH.
Telephone 071 935 0185.

A heart research charity. The foundation can also offer information on self-help groups for people who have recovered from
heart attacks.

First Aid Courses

If you would like to go on a first aid course you can contact
either St John Ambulance for England and Wales, St Andrew's
Ambulance Association, or the British Red Cross. You will find
the contact numbers in your telephone book or the *Yellow
Pages*.

The Foundation for the Study of Infant Deaths

35 Belgrave Square, London, SW1X 8QB.
Telephone 071 235 1721 (24-hour Cot Death Helpline).

The foundation was established in 1971 to raise funds for
research into the causes and prevention of cot death and to give
support to bereaved families. It also acts as a centre of information for parents and professionals.

The Institute for the Study of Drug Dependence (ISDD)

1 Hatton Place, Hatton Garden, London, EC1N 8ND.
Telephone 071 430 1993.

Has information on research about solvents and other drugs.

The Standing Conference on Drug Abuse (SCODA)
at the above address, has information about agencies around
the country where drug and solvent misusers and their families
can get help.
Telephone 071 430 2341.

National Asthma Campaign

Providence House, Providence Place, London, N1 0NT.
Telephone 071 226 2260.

Asthma Helpline
0345 01 02 03 (calls charged at local rates).

The helpline is staffed by trained asthma nurses and offers
advice and counselling to asthma sufferers and their carers. It is
open weekdays from 1–9 p.m.

Re-Solv

The Society for the Prevention of Solvent and Volatile
Substance Abuse
30A High Street, Stone, Staffs, ST15 8AW.
Telephone 0785 817885.

This is a charity solely concerned with solvent misuse. It pub-
lishes leaflets, booklets and videos and has information about
local agencies who can help.

Royal Society for the Prevention of Accidents (RSPA)

The Priory, Queensway, Cannon House, Birmingham, B4 6BS.
Telephone 021 200 2461.

The Stroke Association

CHSA House, 123–127 Whitecross Street, London, EC1Y 8JJ.
Telephone 071 490 7999.

Funds research into the causes and better treatment of strokes
and provides practical help for sufferers and their families.

AUSTRALIA

The Child Accident Prevention Foundation of Australia
10th Floor, 123 Queen Street, Melbourne, Victoria 3000
Telephone 613 670 1319

The Commandery in Western Australia
298 Wellington Street, Perth, Western Australia 6000

National Asthma Campaign
PO Box 360, Woden, ACT 2606
Telephone 06 295 3777

National Safety Council of Australia
322 Glenferry Road, Malvern, Victoria 3144
Telephone 03 824 8822

CANADA

Canadian Heart Foundation
Suite 1200, 1 Nicholas Street, Ottawa, Ontario K1N 7B7
Telephone: 613 237 4361

Parents of Allergic and Asthmatic Children
Box No 4500, Edmonton, Alberta TEE 6K2

The Priory of Canada
312 Laurier Avenue East, Ottawa, Ontaria K1N 6P6
Telephone 613 236 7461

hangovers:
    alcohol, abuse of *129–31*;
    first aid *129*;
    prevention *130*;
    safe drinking *131*;
    signs and symptoms *129*
head: bumps on *59*;
    gashes on *229–30*;
    headaches *133*;
    injuries *132*
headaches: *133*;
    migraine *161–2*
headlice: effect of *134*;
    first aid *134–5*;
    prevention *135*;
    signs and symptoms *134*
heart attacks: cause *135*;
    diet *138–9*;
    exercise, lack of *140–1*;
    fats, risk of *138*;
    first aid *136*;
    heart failure, and *141*;
    high blood pressure *139–40*;
    men and women, proportion in *142*;
    prevalence of *135–6*;
    prevention *137–41*;
    signs and symptoms *136*;
    smoking, risk of *137*
heart disease: *137*
heart failure: *141*
heart massage: adult, for *14*;
    child, for *15*;
    when required *13*
heat illnesses: first aid *143*;
    prevention *143*;
    signs and symptoms *142*;
    strenuous exercise, effect of *142*;
    types of *142*
Hepatitis B: *235*

hernias: cause *143*;
    first aid *144*;
    hiatus *143–4*;
    rupture *143*;
    signs and symptoms *144*
heroin: *103*
hiccups: *144–5*
high blood pressure: *139–40*
HIV: first aid, risk in *235*
Home Accident Surveillance System: *4*
home: accidents in *3*
hospital: driving patient to *5*
housemaid's knee: *145*
hyperventilation: *173*
hypothermia: first aid *146–7*;
    meaning *145*;
    outdoor expeditions, in *147*;
    prevention *147*;
    signs and symptoms *146*
hysteria: *148*

I

ibuprofen: *39*
immunisation:
    German measles, against *124–5*;
    Hib vaccine *150–1*;
    measles, against *159*;
    mumps, against *167*;
    programme *149–51*;
    timetable *150*;
    whooping cough, against *214*
immunisation reactions:
    first aid *150*;
    signs and symptoms *149–50*;
    small risk of *149*
impalement: *151–2*
indigestion: first aid *153*;
    prevention *153*;
    symptoms of *152*
infected wounds: *153–4*
influenza: *154–5*

245